Choose the Sex of Your Baby

naturally

Choose the Sex of Your Baby

naturally

by Pat Buie, B.Sc.N., B.Ed.

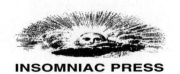

INSOMNIAC PRESS

Edited by Jan Barbieri
Copy-edited by Pamela Murray
Designed by Mike O'Connor

National Library of Canada Cataloguing in Publication Data

Buie, Pat 1953–
   Choose the sex of your baby naturally

Includes bibliographical references.
ISBN 1-894663-02-0

1. Sex preselection. I. Title.

QP279.B84 2001   613.9'4   C2001-930397-1

The publisher gratefully acknowledges the support of the Canada Council, the Ontario Arts Council and Department of Canadian Heritage through the Book Publishing Industry Development Program.

Printed and bound in Canada

Insomniac Press, 192 Spadina Avenue, Suite 403,
Toronto, Ontario, Canada, M5T 2C2
www.insomniacpress.com

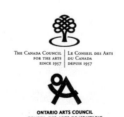

THE CANADA COUNCIL | LE CONSEIL DES ARTS
FOR THE ARTS | DU CANADA
SINCE 1957 | DEPUIS 1957

ONTARIO ARTS COUNCIL
CONSEIL DES ARTS DE L'ONTARIO

To my husband, Neil, who believed that more people should have the chance to be as fortunate as we.
To my children, Jennifer, Erin and Matthew, who are all we ever wanted.

Acknowledgements

My husband, Neil, for suggesting that the knowledge we'd learned and the success we'd had in planning our son should be shared with other parents.

My children, for putting up with my taking over the computer for long periods and inopportune times to write and edit the book.

The many people who have corresponded with me, for letting me know that the information on how to determine the sex of a baby was helpful and valued. The wonderful success stories and letters of appreciation were inspiring.

My editor, Jan Barbieri, for her encouragement, expertise, suggestions and hard work in helping me to improve the manuscript and making this publishing experience so rewarding.

Mike O'Connor, my publisher, for his faith in the topic and in me.

Contents

Foreword

Choosing to become a parent is a monumental moment in a person's life; choosing the sex of your child must be an equally important and well-thought-out decision. Pat Buie provides a great outline to walk people through this detailed process of sex selection. In a logical, step-by-step method, she discusses the rationale for sex selection, reviewing both the history and the various reasons for trying to influence a child's gender prior to conception, providing the basis for a couple to begin an open and honest dialogue prior to pregnancy. Most importantly, she emphasizes acceptance of the child, regardless of gender.

But *Choose the Sex of Your Baby Naturally* not only guides you through the whys of sex selection, it also navigates the hows. In an easy-to-understand, organized manner, Pat provides an educational explanation of genetics, fertility and conception. Anyone can understand her descriptions for determining ovulation—information that is very helpful for any couple wanting to become pregnant, even those not interested in sex determination. The examples of basal body temperature measurements are extremely helpful, and the steps for naturally selecting the sex of your child by determining a woman's fertile peroids, timing intercourse appropriately, and using specific positions are clear, concise and supported by a copious amount of anecdotal data.

The greatest strength of this book is its variety of options: whether or not to choose to have a child, how to choose the sex of your baby and even which method of sex selection to choose. All sides of the issues are addressed in an unbiased manner, ensuring that the emo-

tionally charged and controversial topic of sex selection is
covered in an ethically responsible way.

Gillian Yeates,
B.A., M.D., F.R.C.S.C. (Obstetrics and Gynecology)

Introduction

Since you have just begun reading this page, you must be curious in finding out if you really *can* determine the gender of your child. For centuries, people have dreamed and inquired as you have—you're not the first, nor will you be the last, to ask this question. The good news is, the answer is *yes!* You can choose the sex of your baby by using a method that is non-invasive, drug-free, inexpensive and completely natural. Simply by understanding the workings of the male and, particularly, the female reproductive systems, you will learn not only how to plan your pregnancies, but how to time intercourse to increase your chances of conceiving either a girl or a boy. The method described in this book can help to dramatically increase your chances of conceiving a boy by greater than 80 percent, and slightly less than 75 percent of conceiving a girl.

Today, many couples use natural family planning as a method of preventing or planning pregnancies. Couples who use this method are very knowledgable about and aware of their own fertility. In particular, they are able to determine the times in the woman's menstrual cycle when she is most likely to conceive or get pregnant. To ascertain when she is most fertile, she observes and records the signs and symptoms that her body displays. Her fertile period would be a bracket of time before and after ovulation. With this information, a couple could plan to have intercourse when conditions were favorable for conceiving a baby.

The theory of natural sex selection combines this knowledge with an understanding of the genetic and physical differences between the sperm that produce females and the sperm that produce males: how long they live, how fast they can move through the reproductive tract and what conditions are most favorable for either type of sperm. With this knowledge, the couple can time intercourse for when conditions are favorable for either the male or female sperm, enabling the couple to then plan not only the pregnancy, but the *sex* of their child. And, just as parents are often interested in family planning, they are as likely to be interested in the potential of planning the sex of their children.

When I worked as a public health nurse I taught prenatal classes for several years and made Well Baby visits to new parents. One of the questions that was often asked was, did I know how to make a girl or boy baby? One of the books that I used as a reference when I taught natural family planning was *The Billings Method, Controlling Fertility Without Drugs or Devices*. In one paragraph, the book refers to a study that described the ability of couples to predetermine the sex of their baby. Admittedly, the questions asked of me and the notation itself sparked my curiosity. Through further research, I learned of a specific method, which I describe and expand upon in this book. It is not new-age quackery—it's a time-tested, reliable method based, in large part, on the scientific research of Landrum B. Shettles, a recognized fertility expert.

But the information I found on natural sex selection was often unclear or difficult to follow. After I had finished reading Shettles and other resources, it was evident that an easy-to-read book was needed for couples who wished to readily understand the concept of natural sex selection, without having to read a textbook. I felt that the book should include everything they would need to know in order to learn about their fertility, to understand how to choose the sex of their baby and to feel confident in the method and their ability to succeed. *Choose the Sex of Your Baby Naturally* is just that. It is written for both women and men, discussing the involvement and importance of the role of both partners in the venture. The book covers the basics of anatomy, reproduction, fertility, conception, and possible fertility problems for both men and women. Unlike other books on sex preselection, I describe and illustrate each of three main techniques that work the best to determine exactly when a woman ovulates, and teach you how to interpret the various signs of fertility in the body. My technique for natural sex selection takes you step-by-step through the process, giving you examples and opportunities to practice what you've learned.

Before you start this or any other fertility or sex selection method, it is very important to realize that you must be prepared for a child of either sex. For this reason, before proceeding, I ask of you three things:

1. Examine honestly your reasons for wanting a son or daughter.
2. Decide if these motives are valid—are you being realistic? Think down the road, or to the future.
3. Most importantly, determine whether you want a baby, whatever the sex.

Once you have sorted out your thoughts on these three issues, read on. Even if you have decided not to proceed with another pregnancy, you will be enriched with the knowledge to be gained from this book. Whatever your purpose, I congratulate you on taking a first step in learning more about the wondrous workings of your body and your personal health.

Author's Note

Like most birth control and fertility methods, nothing is 100 percent foolproof. Using the method described in this book will not guarantee that you will have the boy or the girl baby you so desire. If you are not prepared to accept the "other" sex, then perhaps you should not try at all.

However, if you know you will be happy with either sex, and would like to increase your odds dramatically, read on.

PART ONE

Making the Choice:
What is Sex Selection?
Is It Right for Us?

It is necessary to understand the idea of sex selection and what it is all about before you can decide whether it is right for you. In this section, Chapter 1 outlines the history and development of natural sex selection, from the early Greeks to the late-twentieth century. This chapter also covers the unnatural methods of sex selection so you may understand all of the aspects of this idea, allowing you to make a complete and informed decision to determine what's best for you as parents. Chapter 2 discusses the many reasons why people seek to choose their baby's sex, with personal examples taken from letters on the subject that I have received over the past few years. This chapter also examines the ethics and consequences of sex selection.

Having read the information in these chapters, you will be better able to decide if preselecting the sex of your child works for you—if it fits your moral, ethical or religious codes.

Chapter 1
A History of the Development of Sex Selection

Theories of Early Science and Folklore

For centuries, mankind has been trying to find ways of determining the sex of a child prior to conception. Whether they worked or not, the earliest methods were what we consider natural because they did not rely on invasive or surgical techniques. Aristotle (384–322 BC) believed that several forces of nature were responsible: increased vigor would make semen (the male reproductive fluid) more powerful; the couple had a greater chance of having a female if there were a cold, southern wind; and that facing north or a north wind would cause a boy to be conceived. The Greeks also said that the man's lying on his right side during intercourse would produce a male, on his left side, a female. This belief was based on dissections of animals that revealed that some animals had two uteruses. They deduced that because all things just and good came from or to those who were right-handed, lying on the right side during intercourse would produce a male. Conversely, the dominance of the left hand meant one was devious and sneaky, hence having intercourse on the left side would yield a female.

Another Greek philosopher, Anaxagoras (500–428 BC), thought that the man was responsible for producing male offspring. He believed that the right testes had a superior blood supply and therefore produce the "male" semen. The "female" semen, then, would be produced from the left testes. Tying off one or the other testicle would allow the woman to conceive a child of the desired sex.

Hippocrates (460–377 BC), the father of the Hippocratic oath and known for his elaborate theories of reproduction, believed that each testicle was responsible for the particular sex of an offspring, and joined two of the Greek theories. He maintained that tying a string around the "undesired" testicle would produce the preferred result. In addition, he professed that another way to acquire a male child was to have both partners lying on their right sides during intercourse. Again, the right side would yield a male, while the left resulted in a female.

The Hebrew culture offers a more accurate theory. According to folklore, a child's gender depended upon which parent was more passionate at the time of conception. Likewise, the Talmud, the body of ancient texts of Jewish law and legend, maintains that if the woman emits her "semen" (i.e., has an orgasm) before the man, the child would be a boy. Tradition also prescribes that Orthodox Jews abstain from intercourse for the first two weeks of the woman's cycle. Interestingly, this group has a disproportionate number of male offspring. (See Chapter 9 for a discussion of timing intercourse and the role of orgasm in natural sex selection.)

During the Middle Ages, superstition and alchemy played a large role in determining ideas about reproduction. In Germany, the woodsman carried an ax to bed and chanted a "boy chant" to yield a male. With no ax and a "girl chant", he would cause his wife to conceive a female. The Swedes suggested that the bride sleep with a baby boy on the night before her wedding to ensure she would give her new husband a male child. In many countries, the belief was that if the man wished to have a son, either he should have his boots on or his wife should wear men's clothing during intercourse. Another tale suggested that hanging the man's pants on the right or left side of the bed would produce a male or female, respectively. In Austria, the midwife would bury a new mother's placenta (the afterbirth) under a nut tree to ensure her next child would be a boy. Nuts seemed to be very important, because they believed if there were a good crop of nuts, there would be a good "crop" of boys.

More recently, the idea that the woman was responsible for the sex of the child became common. In 1917 it was falsely thought that an egg released from a woman's right ovary would beget a male child, from her left, a female. Believing that the ovaries took turns releasing an egg, the logic ran that the woman could conceive a girl one month or a boy the next. How could they know which month was which? This method was probably used after the first child was born, when they could count back to the month of conception to ascertain the beginning of the pattern for which month made the boy and which made the girl. And, in a similar vein to early Greek ideas about fertility being dictated by natural phenomena was the 1973 book, *Natural Birth Control and How to Choose the Sex of Your Child* by Lynn Schroeder and Sheila Ostrander. In this theory, timing is factor, but so is astrology: they wrote that intercourse needed to be timed in relation to the moon's phases and the position of the stars.

However, mystics, philosophers and doctors have not been the only sources for proposed methods of sex selection. A year or two after a friend of mine had given birth to her third girl, her uncle, a dairy farmer, told her his "recipe" for determining the sex of his calves. If her uncle wanted heifers (females), he would breed the cows early in their cycle. If he wanted bulls (males), he bred them when the cows were just about at the end of their fertile period (right after ovulation). His records of farm births revealed how effectively his "recipe" worked. Shortly thereafter, my friend followed his advice when planning her next child. Just over nine months later, she phoned her uncle to tell him she and her husband had had a son. A modern theory!

Theories from Modern Scientific Research

While many of the earlier theories were true folklore and may have seemed strange, several were on the right track. In fact, both the proscriptions of the Talmud and "recipe" of the dairy farmer are validated by scientific research. Many of the theories about sex determination that have developed over the years have evolved from the modern scientific field of genetics, the science of heredity. Genetics deals with the ways that living organisms are like their parents. In the 1860s, Gregor Johann Mendel, an Austrian monk, discovered that inherited characteristics are carried by tiny particles called genes. His work was confirmed later, when it was discovered that genes are arranged in single file along the chromosomes, the thread-like bodies in the nucleus of a cell. All the chromosomes could be matched into pairs except for two. Edouard van Beneden, in 1883, confirmed these findings: the sex cells (egg and sperm) have half the number of chromosomes that are found in all the other cells of the body. At the beginning of the twentieth century, the zoologist C.E. McClung called the mismatched pair the "sex chromosomes". The smaller one looked like a Y and the larger resembled an X. It was hypothesized that the Y determined the male sex, and the X determined the female sex.

Most of the current theories that have progressed in the last 80 years are thus based upon the premise that there are two types of sperm cells. There is a sperm that bears an X chromosome, resulting in the birth of a female child, and a sperm that carries the Y chromosome of the male child. The egg, however, carries only the X chromosome.

Dr. Shettles and the Late-twentieth Century

Only in the past 40 years have more precise theories of sex determination and sex selection emerged from true scientific research. One of the pioneers in this field is Dr. Landrum Shettles, who was an associate professor of obstetrics and gynecology at the College of Physicians and Surgeons at Columbia University, and the director of research at the New York Fertility Research Foundation. During his fertility research in the 1960s, Shettles discovered that he could distinguish two different sizes and shapes of the sperm he was examining under a microscope. He concluded that they corresponded to the two sexes: the male, or Y-bearing sperm, was small and round, and appeared to move faster than the large, oval-shaped female, or X-bearing, sperm; and this female sperm also appeared hardier or more resilient than the male sperm.

From this data, Dr. Shettles surmised that upon intercourse the male sperm cells move through the woman's reproductive tract faster than the female sperm cells. Thus, if there were an egg about to burst or waiting in the fallopian tubes ready to be fertilized, the faster male sperm would most likely get to the egg first, and hence, a male child would be conceived. However, if intercourse occurred two to three days prior to the egg's release, it would be more likely that the stronger female sperm that could withstand the more acidic environment of the female reproductive tract would outlast the male sperm and reach the egg, and a girl would probably be conceived. Dr. Shettles discusses this theory and the relevant research in his book, *How to Choose the Sex of Your Baby: The Method Best Supported by Scientific Evidence*. Since his book's release in the 1970s, Shettles has continued to be a prominent expert and pioneer in the science of reproduction and female infertility.

Over the years, other researchers have confirmed Dr. Shettles's theory. Dr. Franciszik Benendo's research supported the "timing theory" in the August 13, 1972 issue of *Medical World News*. In 1975, Dr. B. Seguy from France, like Shettles, reported a success rate of almost 80 percent in selecting a male child based on this theory. *Parents* magazine reported in 1981 that Dr. Michael O'Leary, an obstetrician/gynecologist affiliated with the New York Medical Center was using the Shettles method with a 75 percent success rate. Dr. Shiro Sugiyama of Tokyo claimed a 90 percent success rate with the same method.

However, there has been some dissent. E. Whelan, in her 1977 book *Boy or Girl?*, refutes Dr. Shettles's method as she proposes her own theory. Whelan falsely claims that Shettles's data is based upon couples who were using artificial insemination. Whelan loses more credibility throughout the book with several contradictory assertions and inconsitensies in her method. The information becomes confusing to sort out and the book has been questioned by the medical community.

In 1982 Sally Langendoen and William Proctor suggested another theory in *The Preconception Gender Diet*. They indicated that to have a girl, the mother needs a diet high in calcium and low in salt and potassium. For a boy, her diet must be high in salt and potassium and low in calcium and magnesium. This theory of sex selection has generated several conflicts. First, the theory is based on manipulating mineral levels in the female system and, while it has claimed successful results, scientists and doctors are unsure of how this kind of manipulation relates directly to sex determination. Furthermore, Langendoen and Proctor advise the woman wishing to conceive a boy to have a diet high in salt and low in calcium, or to avoid milk and milk products, and advocate the consumption of beer and wine; yet these are not necessarily recommendations that promote an optimum level of health and nourishment, especially for a woman hoping to conceive. This diet is fairly controversial, and is to be investigated only under the watchful eye of one's doctor. I personally don't recommend this diet, but I have included some material on it in Appendix A for your information.

Other Natural Methods

Currently, there are two other natural methods for trying to choose the sex of a baby. The first is by means of astrology and the second is based on an ancient Chinese chart.

1. Choice Through Astrology Can timing the moment of conception around the movement of the moon and stars predetermine the sex of a baby? The answer is yes, according to Dr. Eugene Jonas (pronounced Yohnash), a Czech psychiatrist and gynecologist. In 1956, Dr. Jonas began his research after he found part of an ancient Babylonian-Assyrian text that stated, "Woman is only fertile during a certain phase of the moon." He believed that choosing the hour of conception according to the moon's astrological sign could predetermine the sex of the child. According to astrology, the time of a woman's fertility depends on the recurrence of the angle of the sun and the moon that occurred at the woman's own birth. For example, if the woman were born during the time of a new moon, she would be fertile during the time of the new moon. If she were born with the sun and moon at a 50-degree angle, then she would be fertile when the sun and the moon were at a 50-degree angle each month, and also for a period on each side of this celestial positioning, no matter what was happening in her menstrual cycle. In this theory, the sex of the child depends on the position of the moon at the time of conception. Conception at the moment when the moon is in a masculine, or yang, sign of fire and air will result in a boy. Likewise, if the moon is in a feminine, or yin, sign of earth and water, conception will result in a girl. The moon changes signs approximately every two and a half days. Uniting the desired moon sign with the lunar cycle to insure conception can take several months.

To understand more about this method, you should probably consult an astrologist. However, as I mentioned in an earlier section of this chapter, there is also a book on the subject that claims a 98 percent success rate using the moon sign selection. *Astrological Birth Control* was written by Sheila Ostrander and Lynn Schroeder and was the work that first brought Jonas's theory to the attention of Western culture.

2. Choice By Way of the Ancient Chinese The Ancient Chinese Birth Gender Chart claims a 99 percent accuracy in predicting the sex of a child. Apparently the chart was buried in a tomb near Beijing for 700 years and is now being kept in the Institute of Science in Beijing. The chart states that you can predict the sex of your unborn child if you know the month the child was conceived and the age of the mother at the time of conception. In order to pres-elect the sex of your child, you could probably use these same facts in determining the right month to have intercourse to have a baby of the desired sex, or so the theory goes.

When I consulted the chart, it was correct for my first child, a girl, and my third, a boy. However, it predicted that my second daughter was to have been a boy. Visit *http://mypage.direct.a/j/jfeng/gender.htm* to learn more about this ancient resource.

The Unnatural Methods

Over the years, several so-called unnatural methods of sex selection have been developed. By "unnatural" I mean approaches which involve human interference that is artificial or invasive. The methods can be broken down into pre-fertilization and post-fertilization techniques. The first pre-fertilization method, which is very expensive, is called sperm selection. The method involves separating the male from the female sperm and then using the companion procedures of artificial insemination or in vitro fertilization in order to fertilize the egg with the desired sperm. Although the techniques of artificial insemination and in vitro are often used by couples experiencing infertility, their use in combination with sperm selection as a means for sex selection is not presently a common practice.

The second method falls into the category of a post-fertilization technique. It involves determining the sex of the conceived child and acting upon this knowledge, either by aborting the fetus or even killing the child after it is born if it is not the desired sex. Post-fertilization sex selection practices are not generally accepted in Western culture, and are often illegal. I mention them only in service of completeness of this information, and because, unfortunately, they do exist in some parts of the world.

Unnatural Pre-fertilization Methods

1. Selection Through Sperm Separation The first unnatural method of sex selection begins with the separation of the male and female sperm. In the 1980s, a man by the name of Dr. Ronald J. Ericsson was using a method he had developed to separate sperm. The method became widely used throughout the United States and several other countries around the world. In the most recent version I was able to find of Ericsson's method for producing male babies, diluted semen is spread over a 10 percent solution of serum albumin derived from human blood (albumins are blood proteins manufactured by the liver). After 45 minutes have elapsed, the sperm that have been allowed to swim down into the albumin are extracted by means of a centrifuge, which spins the serum. The sperm are then placed on a two-layer preparation where they remain for one hour. The bottom layer is more dense. The few sperm that penetrate that layer are usually Y-bearing, or male, sperm.

In 1987 it was reported that a Japanese doctor, Rihachi Iizuka, had developed a different method. Using a procedure adapted from a method used to sort blood cells of slightly different composition, he separated sperm into layers, one 95 percent female and the other 85 percent male. The difference in the DNA composition (the arrangement and amount of genetic material, or chromosomes, in a cell) of the male and female sperm was noted on the basis that the male sperm contained 2.8 percent less genetic material than the female sperm. Again, the diluted semen was laid on top of a gel with layers of increasing density and then centrifuged for 20 minutes. Similar to Ericsson's findings, the rate at which the types of sperm moved through the layers differed. However, in Iizuka's method, the female sperm moved slightly faster than the males. Dr. Iizuka stated that after centrifuging, 85 percent of the sperm in the top layer were found to be male and 95 percent of those in the bottom layer were female. Male sperm could be identified by a spot within their nucleus that would glow after being stained with a fluorescent compound.

The *New York Times* reported on September 9, 1998 that the Genetics and IVF Institute, a fertility clinic in

Fairfax, Virginia, had developed another sorting method based on the amount of DNA contained in sperm. Using a DNA detector, researchers were able to sift sperm to produce samples in which 85 percent of the cells were female sperm. They also managed a sample where they obtained 65 percent male sperm. Now, another method was available to complete the first step of this procedure for predetermining the sex of a baby.

With the ability to separate sperm intact, there needs to be a way of getting the right sperm to the egg. Two methods respond to this need: artificial insemination and in vitro fertilization.

2. Artificial Insemination Once the sperm of the desired sex have been obtained, the next step is artificial insemination (AI), the process whereby sperm is placed into the vagina by means other than sexual intercourse. This second step is fairly invasive. Using a device such as an ordinary barrel plunger syringe, the fertile sperm are placed deep into the woman's vagina near the cervix at her most fertile time, when she is ovulating. Sometimes the sperm are deposited as far as the cervical canal or even directly into the uterus using a sterile catheter. Following the insemination, the woman lies quietly on her back, with her buttocks raised to keep the sperm near the cervix.

The statistics seem to reveal that pregnancy rates average 15 to 20 percent for the first insemination. The cumulative probability of pregnancy increases with each cycle with 75 percent of women achieving pregnancy by six months. It was reported that using AI as a method for obtaining the desired sex is about 75 to 80 percent successful for getting the boy and about 65 percent for a girl. However, the Genetics and IVF Institute reported that 13 out of 14 couples requesting a female were successful, but that producing males was more difficult. In 1987, Ericsson reported that efforts to produce boys were about 85 percent successful, girls were about 73 percent. The Japanese technique, developed by Dr. Iizuka, reported close to 100 percent success when the girl was sought.

When reports of Dr. Iizuka's procedure was used for preselecting a baby's gender were first released in Japan, they unleashed a furor: the ethical debate was on. Is the procuring of sperm of the desired sex and the use of AI to predetermine the sex of a baby ethically and morally right? Its artificiality may be the reason why so many are against it. Some may feel that it requires too many steps and "interferences" with the normal happenings of the both the male and the female bodies: semen collection, multi-step sperm separation and the invasive technique of artificial insemination.

3. *In Vitro Fertilization* In vitro fertilization (IVF) is a procedure that involves extracting eggs from the female and sperm from the male and putting them together in a laboratory dish to facilitate fertilization. The fertilized eggs are transferred several days later into the female's uterus where it is hoped that implantation and the normal embryo development in a pregnancy will take place. This procedure was initially developed in the 1970s as a means of treating women whose infertility was caused by damaged or blocked fallopian tubes. The technique involves four stages.

    • *Ovarian stimulation and monitoring* In the first stage, medication causes several eggs to mature. An egg must be mature before it can be fertilized, and ovarian stimulation ensures that at least some of the eggs retrieved will be able to be fertilized and, possibly, result in a pregnancy.

• *Egg retrieval* During the second stage, the doctor attempts to remove as many eggs as possible to increase the chances of fertilization of the eggs.

• *Fertilization* Approximately two hours before the eggs are retrieved, a semen sample is collected from the male. The sperm are "washed", or processed to separate-out the strongest, healthiest and most active sperm in the sample. The sperm are then placed together with the eggs and incubated at the same body temperature as the female.

• *Embryo transfer* After about 48 hours, the fertilized egg, now called a zygote, is transferred into the female's uterus by means of a catheter inserted through the vagina and cervix.

With IVF the rate of success or delivery of live babies is about 20 percent, usually higher in women younger than the age of 40.

Unnatural Post-fertilization Methods
1. *Abortion* A post-fertilization method of sex selection involves either ultrasound or the procedure of amniocentesis and, after serious decision-making, abortion, a topic which itself is ethically controversial.

The first objective is to identify the sex of the fetus. It is possible to observe the developing fetus by means of ultrasound technology whereby high frequency waves are transmitted through the mother's abdominal wall. The sound waves bounce off tissues of different densities and are recorded, creating an image of the fetus on a computer monitor, whereby the sex can be identified. (This method is fairly accurate; however, I do know of times the assessment of the sex by ultrasound was incorrect, in other words, the parents were told they were having a girl, and a boy was born or vice versa.) When amniocentesis is performed, a needle is carefully inserted through the woman's belly into her uterus, and cells in the amniotic fluid (the fluid the fetus is "floating" in) are withdrawn. An examination of the chromosomes of these cells can then determine whether the fetus is a boy or a girl.

Ultrasound and amniocentesis are commonly used in many women's pregnancies to check the development and health of the fetus. However, with this knowledge, a couple could decide either to terminate the pregnancy because the fetus was not the desired sex or to continue the pregnancy. Aborting a fetus just because it is the "wrong"sex is even more of a legal and moral issue than the topic of abortion alone, and one that is definitely against my own ethical principles.

2. *Infanticide* Infanticide is the murder of a newborn child. It is a practice used in some cultures that promote the predominance of one sex over another and/or those that limit the number of children per couple, usually to one child. Clearly, this is illegal in most, if not all countries, and it is also against my own principles.

In Support of Natural Sex Selection

Word of mouth was the source of "expert" advice I received when my husband and I decided that we'd like to have another baby and to try for a boy. I later discovered that this advice was, essentially, Dr. Shettles's method. And, yes, we conceived our boy. In looking back at my ovulation pattern, our two daughters confirm the method: they should have been girls. Not only do my husband and I attest to this kind of natural sex selection, but as I was researching and writing this book, five of my friends and acquaintances who attempted natural sex selection were rewarded with the desired sex of their baby using the method that I have tailored and outlined here. What's more, in the last seven years, approximately 50 couples that had heard of my technique through friends, nurses, and other couples, have personally contacted me to let me know that they had used the same method. Of those 50, only four were not successful in conceiving the gender of their choice. Furthermore, one of the couples had written that, although they were not successful, they had made some mistakes and their child was the sex that the method advocated, in other words, the child confirmed the method. Of the other three couples, I was not able to ascertain whether they possibly made a mistake or did not follow the method properly. Whatever their response, the 46 success stories are certainly impressive.

You, the reader, may have found other methods of gender preselection that I have not mentioned. That's great! I thank those who sent me the results of their research on the topic for my own information. I hope it has made for interesting and provocative reading. Now that you understand what sex selection is and the various methods used, you should examine the reasons and consequences making this choice may have for you.

Chapter 2
Should We Choose the Sex of Our Baby?

Some Reasons Couples Choose

From 1979 to 1983, I worked as a public health nurse for the Simcoe County Health Unit in Ontario, Canada. During this time, I taught prenatal classes and worked in a family planning clinic. After the birth of my first daughter, I continued to teach prenatal classes in the evenings for another eight years. Many times I was asked the question, "Do you know how I could have either a boy or a girl?" At that time I had no idea, but I found the question fascinating. Everyone who had asked me already had had at least one child. Most people, it seemed, just wanted to have one of each sex, although one couple told me that they were so enjoying their daughter that they really wanted to have another girl. After we had had our first child, my husband and I also became quite interested in finding out if there was a way of preselecting a child's sex. Our reasons for doing so were similar to those expressed by many others. For us, we wanted the experience of raising a son.

Due to our success, I generated a booklet detailing my technique. Since then, I have received numerous, letters from people interested in the subject, many of whom expressed their reasons for desiring a child of a particular sex.

Sometimes the reasons were as simple as those of my husband's and mine.

I am a 30-year-old mom with two wonderful daughters—my first will be five years old in November and my second will be

one year old in September. I've entertained thoughts about hav-
ing a third. Although, I wouldn't be disappointed if I had
another girl, it would be nice if we had a boy. —J.S.

My husband and I have two wonderful sons and are planning
a third child. We would love to have a daughter and thought
this would be worth a try. —M.V.

I am the mother of two wonderful little girls. With my first
pregnancy, I wanted a girl really badly. With the second, of
course, I wanted a little boy. I had another girl who is just
great. God has truly showed me that I can love two girls just as
much as loving a girl and a little boy. But there is always that
wonder of what it would be like to have a son. —D.F.

Is the question being asked much more today than in
yesteryear? One hundred years ago, the sizes of families
were much larger. Children were often needed to help the
family sustain itself at home or to be sent out to work.
Because society was lacking in our modern medical
knowledge and the access to vaccines, there was an
increased probability that a child would not make it past
the age of five. For the above reasons, couples had more
children and hence more chances of having children of
both sexes and less of a need or desire to choose a specific gender. We know from history that people did ask the
question and desired to find the answer, but perhaps
because of shyness, politeness, lack of knowledge about
reproduction itself, or for moral reasons, it was not such
an up-front topic for discussion. Now, infant mortality
has drastically declined as children usually live past the
age of five. With couples having fewer children, the sex
selection question is more prevalent.

Other reasons for sex selection can be grouped into

two general categories: desire and necessity. The reasons range from a desire to feel complete as a family or perhaps a desire to please others, and can be rooted in cultural beliefs and stereotypes. And quite often the reasons for sex selection can be serious, stemming from economic considerations or taking into account heredity and serious medical conditions.

Desire

1. *Completing the Family* In her book *Boy Or Girl?*, Elizabeth Whelan discusses commonly expressed reasons for wanting either a boy or a girl. She writes that couples most often mentioned wanting to have at least one child of either sex in order to feel more complete as a family. By having a boy and a girl, they would have the experience of raising children of both sexes, and each partner could enjoy a child who is the same gender as himself or herself. Some of the letters I've received express a similar idea.

I am the privileged mother of three wonderful girls (my youngest is four months old). I know it's a little soon but my husband and I would really like to try one more time for a boy. Our family, as complete as it already sounds, would be absolutely complete with a son. I am the eldest of four daughters and one brother, who is the youngest. Our lives would definitely not have been enriched if my brother were never born. —E.S.

I have two daughters and one son. I would like to have another child. I'm hoping to have another son to balance out my family. —B.B.

Great to finally hear some info… I'm the proud mom of three beautiful boys, but really feel outnumbered by all these men in my life! —C.M.

2. *Pleasing Others* Sometimes couples have written to me expressing a desire to please others by having a child of a particular sex.

I have two girls and we'd like to have a third child. If we have a girl, that will be fine. The important thing is that they are healthy! But it would be nice if we had a boy. My older daughter says that now that she has a little sister, she'd like a little brother. And I think it would be great for my husband, in the sense that he could do father-son things. I'd like to give him a son. —V.H.

I also would like a boy for my husband and for both of our parents. They have only granddaughters. —K.P.

It is exciting to think that I could have a little girl of my own. My husband has three nephews, and I have two. I don't have any sisters and my mother died suddenly when I was seven months pregnant with my first son. I was very close to my mother and was devastated by her death: we were best friends. I now have a void in my life that I need to fill with a little girl of my own. My mother left me with a beautiful heritage that I wish to continue with my daughter. For my mother, for me, I hope to have a baby girl. —S.L.

3. *Cultural and Societal Considerations* Another possible reason that people inquire about ways of predetermining the sex of their child is related to culture or beliefs. In history, of course, dowries often had to be provided for daughters—rather expensive if one had many girl babies! Then, of course, there exists the traditional desire for a

male heir, still a pressure for some. (Look at the world's rejoicing when Diana, Princess of Wales, produced William, and then Harry, "the Heir and the Spare".) Some cultures in the world still genuinely desire a boy over a girl, and often a female has little or no value. China's well-known policy limits families to one child; generally a boy is preferred. Although these factors are not common in Western society, they can still be real pressures for immigrant families who have settled in Western culture.

I am from India, married with a three-and-a-half-year-old daughter... and am eager that my next child be a son. As you know, in India, sons are preferred. —P.S.

I am a new bride. My husband is from India and, of course, his parents have let me know how much they are looking forward to their first grandson. —M.C.

There are many more reasons why couples look for information on determining their baby's sex. Some have expressed the desire to have a particular sex first, which is often linked to stereotypical roles. For example, an older male could protect a younger child, or an older female could help care for younger siblings. Some people prefer having a son so that he can carry on the family name or so that the father will "feel more like a man", having sired a male. Others wish to have a daughter because she would be "someone to take care of"—again the stereotypical feeling that a female is weaker than a male or fragile and therefore needs to be looked after more than the male. Or perhaps a daughter is desired because it is exciting to be a female in today's times!

Necessity

1. Economic Limitations Planning a family has always included economic factors. As mentioned, a hundred years ago, children were an economic asset to the family, needed to help at home or in the workplace. However, today things have changed. The cost of living and the cost of raising a child have made large families difficult to sustain. Children also remain with their parents often well into their twenties, and so have become an increased economic liability. Couples often can only afford one, or two, or maybe three children, so sex selection may become an important part of their family planning.

My husband and I have a beautiful three-year-old daughter. We are both working and will always have to. We would like to have one more child, and would really like to have a son. —I.R.

My husband and I want to have a baby. Because we feel we can only afford to raise on child, I really want to have a boy. —S.C.

My husband and I have one daughter who is two and know we will only be able to afford raising two children. We would really like to have another daughter because they can share clothes and also a room since we live in a two-bedroom house. —G.O.

2. Medical Reasons Finally, parents may have serious medical reasons for wanting to have only female or male children. The cause is usually a genetic illness or disease that might be inherited by the child.

I am very interested in this subject because a genetic disorder runs in my family. My grandmother and my mom both had an affected male baby. Both boys were severely mentally challenged. My uncle died at age five. My brother died when he was

15. It is a disorder that is carried on the X chromosome and I am not sure if I am a carrier or not. A genetic counselor determined that my mother and grandmother were both carriers of the defective X and, in turn, could potentially affect all males conceived. We were also told that, since my brother and uncle had both died, it was like finding a needle in a haystack to identify the problem area on the X chromosome.

I have a 50 percent chance of having an affected male child. To make a long story short, my husband and I would like to start a family and we are interested in having a female child.
—N.P.

Medical reasons like the one above often center around a defective gene on the X chromosome. When such a condition is present, the male offspring commonly display the disease (see Chapter 5 for a discussion of dominant and recessive genes). An example of an X-linked disease is hemophilia, a condition where there is an absence or malfunction of clotting factors in the blood, causing a tendency to bleed easily from minor injuries, with great difficulty in stopping the bleeding. A famous case of hemophilia is that of the little Grand Duke Alexis (1904–1918) who inherited the disease from his mother, Empress Alexandra, wife of Nicholas II, the last czar of Russia.

My husband and I have two wonderful boys but we would like to try for a girl. My youngest son has hemophilia and caring for him and seeing what he will have to live with has really made me think twice about having any more children. —S.M.

A second example of an X-linked disease is Duchenne's muscular dystrophy. Muscular dystrophy causes muscles to become weak and to waste away. It usually affects the muscles that move bones. When a family has a history of either this disease or hemophilia, a female child is often desired.

Finally, the health of the mother, and the subsequent risk to her health because of a pregnancy, may be another medical consideration. If a woman has a history of a particularly difficult pregnancy, labor or period following the birth of a child, or if her own health will be put at risk by more than one more pregnancy, she may be advised that she can only have one more child. Thus, because of medical considerations, the couple may be looking at gender preselection.

Positive and Negative Consequences of Sex Selection

Although we may want the choice, the question still remains, should we do it? Should we predetermine the sex of our children? What are the positive and negative consequences of such knowledge, especially if applied to a whole culture?

An interesting book on this subject is called *Sex Selection in Children*, edited by Neil Bennett. One chapter by John C. Fletcher, entitled "Ethics and Public Policy— Should Sex Choice be Discouraged?" discusses some of the possible consequences of predetermining the sex of a child. Based on Fletcher's essay, I have assembled the following list of possible consequences of both natural and unnatural sex selection.

Potentially Positive Consequences

There is no doubt that there are many positive consequences to the use of sex selection that will not only affect the child, but also the family. Some examples are listed below.

- Life-enhancing benefits can be achieved. Sex-linked diseases such as hemophilia may be avoided.
- If a culture is male-dominated, the conscious choice of a girl child may make her feel especially wanted (i.e., increase her self-esteem or her value in society).
- Family planning (the choosing if and when to have a child) is enhanced.
- A balance in a two-child family can be realized (one girl and one boy).
- Happiness in families may be enhanced.
- Family planning may help control, or slow down, population growth.
- Human understanding of and control over genetics may increase.

Potentially Negative Consequences
As in all issues, there are two sides to the story. Sex selection involves methods and technology that can be used to benefit a majority of the population, but the fear is that it will get out of control or be used for immoral or unethical reasons; in other words it will be used to benefit select groups or to exerise power over others. Many of the common objections concern the unnatural methods of sex selection, and do not necessarily apply to natural methods. The following are potentially negative consequences expressed by some.

- If the process of sex selection is expensive, only a small portion of the population, mainly the rich, will benefit.
- A child's self-esteem could be damaged.
- Overemphasis of sex preferences could encour-

age sexism in society.

• An imbalance of the sex ratio of males to females could result.

• The sex ratio imbalance may result in an increase in conflict between sexes, especially when a higher value is placed on one sex.

• A precedent for eugenics (the science of controlled genetic breeding for desired characteristics in order to improve the human race) could result.

• A possibility of abuse by a totalitarian state may result.

Many of the potentially positive consequences of sex selection were addressed previously in this chapter. But some of the negative issues raise questions themselves, most centering around the question, would there be a disastrous response because we are interfering with nature? Fears of a major change in birth rates (the annual number of live births per 1,000 people), fears of an imbalance (too many of one sex) or fears of a shift in gender value and status in society resulting from sex preference often accompany the topic of sex selection. As suggested earlier, many of these questions—such as the issue of cost and abuse by a governing force—spring from the unnatural methods of sex selection and the technologies they employand are not as relevant to natural sex selection methods. While some of these concerns are valid in terms of unnatural sex selection, the fact remains that these methods are costly, time-consuming, invasive and not practiced by the majority of the population.

In researching this topic, I found the short essays by the many writers in *Sex Selection in Children* most interesting and I use many of their thoughts as well as my own to address the most common concerns surrounding this issue. A response to each of these consequences of sex selection could fill volumes of books; what follows is merely a cursory look at these questions and a starting point for your own discussion.

Dispelling Misconceptions

1. Changes in Birth Rates Would there be a significant change in birth rates? In Western society, the trend towards smaller families is already happening, regardless of the use of sex selection. Time and financial concerns have motivated us to have one to three children. Because of this trend, the total effect that the practice of natural sex selection in family planning will have in altering the number of births per families will be negligible. For those couples who will have a larger number of children in order to achieve a gender balance in the family, the ability to predetermine the sex may decrease the number of children they have. Either way, the drop would be relatively insignificant because the size of our families is already set at a low number.

The story is a bit different when we consider demographics worldwide that generally support larger families. Of course, the ability to choose the sex of a child does not necessarily guarantee that a couple in a culture that values larger families will opt to have a smaller number of children. However, one could argue that the introduction of natural sex selection methods could decrease birth rates, just as the introduction of birth control would. Natural sex selection methods teach a woman how to determine when she fertile and most likely to become pregnant. This understanding gives her more control over her fertility, possibly allowing her to decrease the number of unplanned pregnancies. Furthermore, understanding and using this method successfully in societies where a specific sex is preferred could allow the couple to conceive the sex they desire with the first pregnancy and thus decrease the number of children conceived. Even if the birth rate in these demographics dropped significantly, it would be a help in controlling the alarming and rapidly increasing population problem that the world is facing.

Either way, even if a widespread practice of natural sex selection resulted in a decrease in birth rates, one could argue that a trend toward smaller and more "complete" families would be helpful economically, decrease stress and perhaps increase the quality of life for both children and parents.

2. Upsetting the Gender Balance Would sex selection practices result in an inequality of males to females? A common fear is that a majority of parents will prefer one sex over the other (e.g., everyone will want a boy and no one will want a girl) and thus cause an imbalance in the gender ratio. This outcome is not likely to happen, even with sex selection capabilities. Researchers have confirmed that there would probably be an increase in males, followed by an increase in females a few years later to restore the balance. The effect would probably be similar to what migration or wars have already had in many of the world's societies.

It is conceivable that cultures that traditionally prefer one sex over the other, especially in countries where the number of children allowed is severely limited, would use sex selection to the point of an imbalance in the gender ratio. While this outcome would pose a host of problems, there is a positive side to these types of cultures using sex selection: it could ease harm to "unwanted" children. In the societies in which a boy child is favored,

the cultures are usually those where the female is subor-
dinate to the male, often in developing countries where
there is much poverty and illiteracy. Often the girls are
killed or aborted. For example, an alarm went out in 1982
when it was discovered that some parents in China were
killing female babies. Boys were preferred because of
their economic assets and as a form of security. A boy
could work the fields, carry on Dad's work, and support
his parents in old age. Sex selection in such situations
would thus decrease infanticide and abortions of female
fetuses and diminish the blaming of one of the parents
when the desired sex is not obtained.

3. Altering Gender Status in Society Of course, if, for some
reason, the gender ratio became extremely unbalanced,
there is the possibility for conflict between the sexes,
especially if this conflict were a reflection of destructive
sexist attitudes in society. On the other hand, the result
would not necessarily have to be wholly negative. If, for
example, as a result of sex selection, females were to
decrease in number, their relative position or status could
change: they could become more desirable. Possibly, in
specific cultures, dowries could decrease or be eliminat-
ed—perhaps the male himself would have to pay a
dowry. Or, in jobs traditionally held by women, the smaller number of females may increase the demand for their
services, thereby increasing the wage and the standing of
the female within the family. However, as stated in the
previous section, this kind of outcome is unlikely because
a gender imbalance is unlikely.

4. Self-esteem How can sex selection positively influence
the self-esteem of a child? In a pilot study in *The Secret
Life of an Unborn Child*, Dr. Thomas Verny concluded that

the best factors contributing to the development of a healthy personality were the parents' positive attitude toward the pregnancy and the fulfillment of their desire to have a child of a certain sex. In a situation where the parents weren't happy with the sex of their son or daughter, the child could grow up feeling he or she had failed somehow, simply by perceiving he or she was not what one or both parents wanted. Diana, Princess of Wales, expressed this sentiment herself. She believed her parents had wanted a boy, the heir, and that she was a disappointment to them. Such perceptions can result in withdrawal, antisocial behavior and gender confusion in the child.

On the other hand, it is argued that a child's self-esteem can improve if he or she knows that his or her gender was preferred. An example comes from anthropologist Margaret Mead. One view is that should the sex preference for males diminish, even if it is temporarily, the self-esteem of the female will already have changed for the better. As Mead states, "For the first time in human history, girls would be as wanted as boys." She suggests that as a product of sex selection, a girl would grow up knowing she was truly wanted and not just "settled for."

It is also argued that sex selection could increase not only the child's self-esteem, but the parents' as well. For concerned couples, planning the sex of a child could take away the blame or guilt, or at the very least, a sense of responsibility, from one of the partners. Too bad Henry VIII didn't know more!

If there is any risk that the child would be "rejected" because he or she is not the desired gender, it is my opinion that pregnancy, let alone sex selection, should be reconsidered. As I have stated before, the most important thing is that a parent is ready to accept his or her child, regardless of the child's sex, abilities, and so forth. But it is nice to know that sex selection does have the potential to bolster self-esteem.

5. *Eugenics and Governmental Abuse* There is obviously a reason to fear that sex selection, and more specifically, the unnatural methods, could be abused by a government or totalitarian force in order to shape the population to their own ends; infanticide and abortion have been used for this purpose. For instance, large-scale sex selection could lead to an acceptance and practice of eugenics or to other controversial uses of genetic engineering. It wouldn't be the first time in history that similar abuses have occurred. Unfortunately, potential misuse of technologies that should be used to achieve positive ends (e.g., to improve the quality of human life) is a risk that comes with any form of technology, whether it be new or old, genetic, chemical or mechanical.

Yet, natural sex selection is not really at risk of being abused in this way. First of all, it involves the willing participation of both partners, especially the woman, who must take the time to chart and interpret her menstrual cycle. This would be much more difficult for a government or totalitarian force to track and regulate than it would be for them to employ and enforce an artificial method. Any group who wishes to control the population in this way would probably want to use a method that they could guarantee a specific percentage of success. In natural sex selection, a certain percentage of failure will always result, due to common mistakes in using or understanding the method and from the influence of outside forces. (However, with some of the unnatural methods, the technology could probably be improved to generate a higher percentage of success.) Above all else, natural sex selection is and should really be thought of as an enhancement of family planning.

Moral and Religious Objections

In the last several years, I have received three comments, one in person, one on the phone and one through the mail, to say that choosing the sex of one's child is interfering with Mother Nature or playing God. While I accept that everyone has a right to their own opinions, I also believe that everyone has a right to informed choices. Neither this book nor I promote unnatural or artificial means of achieving the desired sex. However, in my opinion, understanding one's body and making choices based on that knowledge—such as preventing or planning a pregnancy, or possibly increasing one's chances of having a boy or a girl—is not playing God. It is simply working with nature. Ultimately, however, it's your decision.

It is for us to make the effort. The result is always in God's hands. —Mohandas K. Gandhi

Natural Sex Selection: More Good Than Bad

When it is done with the right attitude, and for the right reasons, the benefits of natural sex selection far outweigh any of the disputable negative aspects. The gained knowledge about the human body and process of reproduction; the outcome of happy, satisfied parents with healthier, happier children; and, possibly, the realization of smaller, better-balanced families is well worth the challenging decision. It is a comfort to know that this decision can be made without the moral question of the need to use artificial means such as drugs or genetic engineering.

Nathan Keyfitz, in Bennett's book, *Sex Selection in Children*, summarizes the issue of the consequence of sex selection well:

Stifling this technology would be the same as a primitive moralist urging against the release of the knowledge of "how to make fire" to the public because, although it has great use for warming people and the cooking of food, it may cause a forest fire!

Part Two

The Anatomy and Physiology of Reproduction

You are now aware of the different ways to preselect the sex of your child and also the many reasons for and the consequences of doing so. You know the whys of choosing your baby's sex. Now it is time to learn how.

But first, to understand the basics for determining how to conceive a boy or a girl, one must have a working knowledge of the anatomy and physiology of human reproduction. Chapters 3 and 4 addresses male and female reproductive anatomy, fertility (the ability to produce children) and infertility, complete with diagrams of the reproductive systems. Chapter 5 briefly reviews genetics (how a baby's sex is determined) as well as the process of fertilization, pregnancy and birth.

It's a lot of information. All of it may be new to some of you, some information may be a review for others. It is important that you know the ins and outs of the reproductive systems of both men and women so that when it comes time, you will be able to both chart and interpret your fertility accurately and improve your chances when you try for the girl or the boy. This section is easy to read, and the bodily systems and processes are described so that you will be able to understand quite well how awesome the workings of our bodies are and how miraculous the process of reproduction is.

Chapter 3
Male Anatomy, Fertility and Infertility

Male Anatomy

The male reproductive anatomy is composed of external and internal structures. The external structures, located on the outside of the male's body are the supporting structures of the penis and the scrotum, the glands called the testes and the ducts within those structures. The internal structures are other glands and ducts that transport sperm and seminal fluid. Please refer to the correlating diagrams to better understand the male reproductive anatomy.

Male Reproductive Anatomy (side view)

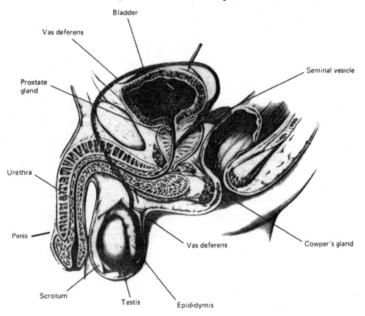

External Structures

1. Penis Composed of spongy, erectile tissue, upon sexual stimulation, the **penis** widens, lengthens and "hardens" as it becomes filled with blood. (The erection also happens as a normal neurological response three or four times a night as the man sleeps.) The penis is the copulatory organ through which the sperm may be introduced into the female's vagina.

2. Scrotum The **scrotum** is a skin-covered pouch suspended from the body. It is divided into two sacs by a septum, or membrane, each sac holding a testis and the **epididymis**.

3. Testes **Testes** is the plural form for two, small, oval-shaped glands, which are the male sexual glands, each of which is called a **testis**. The testes are responsible for the production of **sperm**, the male reproductive cells. Sperm must be kept cooler than the rest of the body, which is why the testes are outside of the body, suspended in the scrotum. The testes also produce the male sex hormone, **testosterone**. Testosterone has many functions, but of major importance is its promotion of "maleness". It causes the secondary sex characteristics of males, such as the development of body hair and the change in body build. Testosterone and other hormones work together in a delicate balance to control sperm production. Any disruption may interfere with sperm development.

4. Seminiferous Tubules The **seminiferous tubules** are tubes located inside each testis, which are responsible for the production of sperm. This function is called **spermatogenesis**, a continuous and complex process in which immature cells gradually develop over 10 to 11 weeks into mature sperm. Once mature, each sperm cell appears tadpole-shaped and is about 2,000 times smaller than the female egg. From puberty on, about 350 to 500 million sperm are produced each day in the seminiferous tubules within the testes. However, it only takes one sperm cell to unite with one egg cell and create a new person.

5. *Epididymis* On the top and the side of each testis is a tightly coiled tube, very small in diameter but approximately 6 meters/20 feet in length, called the **epididymis**. It is a tube through which sperm pass. It also stores the sperm prior to ejaculation and secretes a small amount of seminal fluid.

The Testis

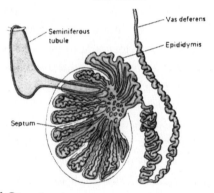

Internal Structures

1. *Vas Deferens* Passing from each testis, through the inguinal canal (a passageway in the groin) and into the abdominal cavity are two ducts. Each duct is called the **vas deferens**, a narrow tube that circles over and down the back of the bladder, carrying the sperm from the testes to the **seminal vesicles**.

2. *Seminal Vesicles* These are coiled or twisted pouches that lie along the lower part of the bladder. Their function

is to produce and release the thick, milky liquid called **seminal fluid** into the vas deferens where it will mix with the sperm. This mixture is called **semen**.

3. Prostate Gland Below the bladder is the donut-shaped **prostate gland**. The prostate secretes a thin alkaline substance that makes up the largest part of the seminal fluid. Because it is alkaline, the substance helps to protect the sperm from the acid present in the male urethra and the female vagina. Acid slows down sperm or, if strong enough, kills it. **Sperm motility** (the sperm's ability to move about directionally, not randomly) is greatest in a neutral or slightly alkaline environment. The secretion from the prostate assists, therefore, in increasing the motility of the sperm.

4. Cowper's Glands Just below the prostate are two small **Cowper's glands**, resembling peas in both size and shape. Like the prostate, these glands secrete an alkaline fluid. A duct approximately 2.5 centimeters/1 inch long connects them to the urethra.

5. Urethra As the vas deferens passes through the prostate it joins into the urethra. The **urethra** is a tube which comes from the bladder and follows a course for about 12 centimeters/8 inches through the prostate and the penis, to the outside of the body. This tube serves two purposes: it is a passageway for eliminating urine from the body and it is a passageway for the expulsion of the reproductive fluid or semen. A small, valve-like muscle at the base of the bladder prevents urine and semen from being in the urethra at the same time. Thus, when semen is exiting through the urethra, urine cannot leave the bladder.

Male Fertility

The man has an important role in reproduction because he provides one half of the new being who is being created. He does so by contributing a sperm cell enveloped in a nourishing fluid. The sperm cell is one of millions that will attempt to find and fertilize the woman's egg.

Usually at some point during sexual stimulation, a man will have an orgasm (the climax of the sexual act) or ejaculation. At the time of **ejaculation**, seminal fluid protecting the sperm cells carries the sperm out of the testes through the vas deferens, along the urethra and out of the penis. During vaginal intercourse, the millions of sperm cells released into the vagina upon ejaculation will start their journey to find the egg.

In theory, each male is always fertile because sperm cells are always being produced. More importantly, sperm can be present in any fluid that leaves the penis: this includes urine and especially the pre-ejaculatory secretion, or "pre-come" that is often on the end of the erect penis. This means that pregnancy can result from genital contact alone, without penetration or ejaculation.

Physical Mechanics

There must be four parts in place, or functioning properly, for the male to be sexually healthy or fertile. A disruption in any of the factors listed below will affect a man's fertility.

1. *Emission* Sperm have to move from the epididymis along through the vas deferens and into the urethra.

2. *Secretions* The seminal fluid must be of the correct consistency and composition for the sperm to be fertile. This

fluid contains nutrients that support sperm metabolism, and is rich in sugar, which provides energy for the sperm to swim.

3. Erection The hardening of the penis is controlled by nerve impulses that dilate certain blood vessels and constrict others so that the erectile tissue in the penis fills with blood. While the penis is erect, ejaculation can occur.

4. Ejaculation This is the process whereby semen is driven along the urethra and out of the body by powerful muscles, some of which are in the penis itself and others that are attached to the urethra.

Sperm Count
Also of great importance in determining a man's fertility is his sperm count. A **sperm count** is the number of sperm ejaculated and the characteristics of the sperm, which include the size, shape and motility of the sperm themselves. A sperm count involves a microscopic analysis of the semen and of the number, health and motility of the sperm in a sample from one ejaculate. The following list gives a more thorough explanation of what is assessed when a sperm count is done.

1. Semen Normally, about 2 to 5 milliliters/0.5 to 1 teaspoon of semen is measured in one ejaculation. If the volume is less than this, the man may not be producing enough seminal fluid. If the quantity is more than 5 milliliters, the seminal fluid may be diluting the sperm too much.

2. Numbers of Sperm The total number of sperm in one

ejaculate should be greater than 40 million per milliliter. If the number is below 20 million, there may be a fertility problem.

3. Sperm Motility At least 40 percent of the sperm should be active and moving.

4. Sperm Appearance Sperm cells are unicellular (one cell) and are made up of a head, a midpiece and a tail. The head holds the genetic information. The midpiece contains fuel and "computer systems" to control movement. The tail-like structure, called the **flagellum**, acts as a kind of propeller or whip to move each sperm forward. At least 65 percent of the sperm should look normal. Any slow, deformed or unusual sperm are defective and should be identified under a microscope.

The Sperm Cell

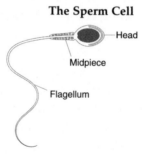

The sperm count for every man is different and often varies depending on environmental conditions. Every male knows the reaction of his genitals when he dives into a cold lake. Sperm do not take kindly to a moderate change in temperature: as cold strikes the body, the genitals are pulled up close to the body for body warmth. Similarly, on a hot summer's day the genitals are very loose and hang away from the body in order to keep as cool as possible. The body naturally looks after itself.

There are methods that will help to keep the sperm count to an optimum level. Keeping the testicles cool by wearing loose underwear and pants and having cool showers can help. Similarly, abstinence will keep the sperm count at an optimum level, allowing it to build up. Moderate physical activity, the curtailing of alcohol and the quitting of smoking and any harmful substances will help boost or keep the count at its optimum. The only exception to the drug rule is caffeine: it has been reported as helping to boost sperm count. A cup of coffee before bed may "wake up" the sperm for the race. As you can see, the environment in which the sperm are produced and stored can greatly influence the sperm count and therefore the male's fertility.

Male Infertility

Male infertility means the inability of the male to produce offspring. In about half the cases of male infertility, the cause can be found. The other half remain a mystery. There are three main causes for male infertility: impaired sperm production, blockages of ducts and channels, and problems with sperm delivery.

Impaired Sperm Production

There are certain factors that can prevent the body from manufacturing and sustaining sperm, resulting in a low sperm count. What follows is a short list of possible interferences.

1. Mumps Mumps is a viral infection, which in the adult male causes damage to the sperm in their initial stage. They cannot mature. Other viruses can also cause damage but usually only temporarily.

2. Undescended Testicles The testes are formed in the abdominal cavity and should descend prior to or at birth. Surgery is needed to correct testicles that have not descended, or damage will be irreversible.

3. Radiation This treatment for cancer kills the immature sperm cells.

4. Use of Drugs Chemicals such as drugs and alcohol can affect the motility of the sperm as well as the count. Cigarette smoke (obviously containing chemicals, too) is also said to affect the sperm count. Certain pharmaceuticals can also damage the newly forming sperm.

5. Age As a man grows older, his sperm count may diminish.

6. Environmental Factors Many environmental factors can influence the production, quality and quantity of the sperm, thereby influencing and/or lowering a man's sperm count. Sperm usually can live for up to five days (one study reported six days) in an optimum environment. As mentioned earlier, heat or cold can kill the sperm, and male (Y-bearing) sperm, it seems, are particularly sensitive to temperature and chemical changes. Thus, clothing that prevents the temperature of the scrotum from being at least one degree lower than body temperature will lower the sperm count. Similarly, extreme physical exercise or a high fever has this same effect because both increase the core body temperature. Finally, sexual activity lowers the sperm count. The more a man ejaculates, the fewer sperm there are in his semen.

Blockages of Ducts and Channels

Structural irregularities or blockages may prevent sperm from joining the seminal fluid and being carried along to the outside of the body. I have included two possible sources of these irregularities.

1. Varicoceles A varicocele is the enlargement of a vein or veins in the testis, occurring most frequently on the left side. It may obstruct circulation to the area causing that part of the testis to wither. It is also possible the increased blood to the area causes an increase in the temperature of the testis. Experts are unsure why it happens.

2. Infections Illnesses such as gonorrhea can cause blockage of ducts.

Problems with Sperm Delivery

Certain conditions can prevent the delivery of semen into the vagina during sexual intercourse. These conditions may include

1. Impotence Impotence is the failure of the ability to have and maintain an erection, thereby preventing sexual intercourse. This inability and failure to be able to ejaculate has many causes, which include nerve injury, drug use, diabetes, stress and psychological factors.

2. Disorders of the Endocrine Glands The endocrine glands release hormones or cause the release of hormones. For example, at puberty, the pituitary gland, at the base of the brain, produces a hormone called follicle stimulating hormone (FSH), which signals the testes to begin producing testosterone.

Other Reasons

In rare cases there are genetic reasons for infertility. Also, diseases such as renal failure, untreated diabetes, alcoholism and malnutrition are all thought to contribute to male infertility. Amazingly, when the body recognizes and identifies problems within, it shuts down systems that are not as necessary or vital to life. Consequently, the reproductive system is one of the first to be affected.

It may seem that male fertility sounds very complicated. Happily, though, the human body is a miracle at work. Without our conscious involvement, everything seems to happen with ease. For the majority of males, infertility is not a concern.

Chapter 4
Female Anatomy, Fertility and Infertility

Female Anatomy

The female anatomy is also divided into the external and internal structures. The external components are obviously those parts which can be seen on the outside of the body. The internal structures, inside the abdomen, are all unique and wondrous in their function of promoting human procreation. Once again, please refer to the correlating diagrams to better understand the female reproductive anatomy.

External Structures

Female Reproductive Anatomy, external

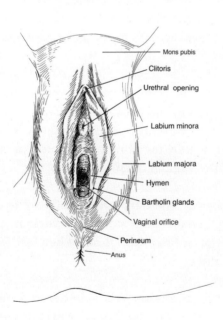

1. *Mons Pubis* The **mons pubis** is a skin-covered padding of fat over a bone called the symphysis pubis. Coarse hairs, called pubic hairs, grow here at puberty.

2. *Clitoris* The **clitoris** is a small organ composed of erectile tissue that may be stimulated during sexual excitement.

3. *Labia Majora* A Latin term meaning "large lips". Covered with skin and hair on the outside and smooth and hairless on the inside, the **labia majora** are composed of fat and many glands.

4. *Labia Minora* A Latin term meaning "small lips", the **labia minora** are found within the labia majora and come together at the midline at the front of the body.

5. *Urethral Opening* The small opening of the urethra (the duct running from the bladder to the outside of the body) is the **urethral opening**. It is located just above the **vaginal orifice**.

6. *Vaginal Orifice* This is the opening of the vagina. In the virginal state, the vaginal orifice is similar in size to the urethral opening because of a constricting border formed by the hymen, a thin membrane stretching across and partly closing the vaginal opening.

7. *Bartholin's Glands* The **Bartholin glands** are two bean-shaped glands, one on either side of the vaginal opening, which secrete a lubricating fluid when the woman becomes sexually excited.

8. *Perineum* The **perineum** is a skin-covered muscular region between the vaginal orifice and the **anus** (the

opening of the rectum). It is affected in childbirth, and its muscles are important for sexual intercourse.

Internal Structures

1. Vagina The **vagina** is a collapsible tube, about 10 centimeters/4 inches long, extending upwards and backwards from the outside of the body to the uterus. It has three functions.

- It passes the menstrual flow from the uterus to the outside of the body.
- It receives the seminal fluid from the male.
- It serves as the lower part of the birth canal, able to expand greatly to allow the baby to be born.

2. Cervix The **cervix** is a thick neck-like structure at the end of the vagina that opens into the uterus. It has an **external os** (Latin for "opening") at the vagina and an **internal os** into the uterus.

Female Reproductive Anatomy, internal (side view)

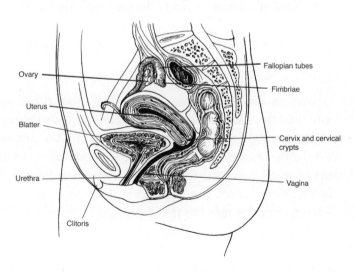

Ovary

Uterus

Blatter

Urethra

Clitoris

Fallopian tubes

Fimbriae

Cervix and cervical crypts

Vagina

3. Cervical Crypts   Within the cervix are the **cervical crypts**, chambers that produce increasing amounts of mucus around the time ovulation. This mucus helps protect the sperm and move them into the uterus.

4. Uterus   Also known as the womb, the **uterus** is a hollow, muscular, pear-shaped organ about 7 centimeters/3 inches in length. The lining of the uterus is called the **endometrium** and usually undergoes cyclic changes each month. The uterus has three important functions.

- It anticipates the arrival of a fertilized egg by thickening and enriching its lining. If fertilization (the union of the egg and the sperm cell) does not occur, then menstruation follows as this spongy lining is discarded.
- When the egg is fertilized, it is called an embryo for the first three months of pregnancy; after that, it is a fetus. The uterus houses the growing embryo, which implants itself into the endometrium and is nourished there.
- Once the fetus is ready to survive outside the mother's body, the muscular uterine wall contracts powerfully and rhythmically to expel its lodger. This is termed labor.

5. Fallopian Tubes and Fimbriae   The **fallopian tubes** run from the upper side of the uterus. They are ducts through which the egg moves from the ovary to the uterus. Fertilization normally occurs in one of these tubes. At the end of each tube are finger-like projections known as **fimbriae** that catch the egg when it emerges from the ovary and pull it into the fallopian tube .

6. *Ovaries* These two female sex glands are shaped like large almonds and are found on either side of the uterus. They perform two functions.

- They produce the eggs, or **ova** (singular **ovum**), which mature and are released into the pelvic cavity near the fimbriae.
- They secrete the female sex hormones. These hormones, **estrogen** and **progesterone**, cause the female secondary sex characteristics, such as the development of body hair and breasts, the change in body build, and the menstrual cycle. A female child is born with all of her underdeveloped eggs, more than she will need in her lifetime!

Female Fertility

The female reproductive system undergoes changes in a cycle that lasts approximately four weeks or one calendar month. This cycle is known as the **menstrual cycle**. The advent of this cycle at puberty signals the beginning of a female's fertile period during her childbearing years. Her reproductive abilities will be dependent upon the proper functioning of the cycle. This amazing process is coordinated by two "control centers", the pituitary gland and the ovaries. At the onset of puberty the pituitary gland begins producing and sending the **follicle stimulating hormone (FSH)** to the ovaries to tell the ovaries to produce mature eggs. FSH and other hormones secreted by the pituitary hormones tell the ovaries what to do and the hormones produced by the ovaries tell the uterus what to do.

The Menstrual Cycle
The menstrual cycle begins the first day of any sign of bleeding and ends the day before the bleeding starts

again in the next cycle. The length of the cycle can vary from woman to woman and from cycle to cycle for the same woman. It is divided into three phases.

1. Pre-ovulatory Phase The **pre-ovulatory phase** begins on the first day that bleeding is noted and ends the day before ovulation. On the first day of the cycle, the pituitary gland releases FSH, causing several eggs in the ovaries to begin to mature. Each egg is wrapped in layers of cells called the **follicle**. As the eggs mature, the developing follicle secretes the hormone **estrogen** in increasing amounts into the blood stream. Estrogen is a hormone that does four things:

- It causes the lining of the uterus to thicken, readying to receive a fertilized egg.
- It also causes the cervical crypts to produce a fertile mucus that will keep sperm alive and create passageways that vibrate to push the sperm up into the uterus.
- It travels back through the blood to the pituitary gland, causing it to release the **luteinizing hormone (LH)**.

Female Reproductive Anatomy, pre-ovulatory phase (front view)

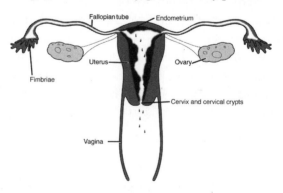

— 70 —

• Finally, the estrogen effects a change in the position of the uterus, causing the cervix to move up in the vaginal canal, to soften and to open wider.

2. *Ovulation* The second phase in the menstrual cycle is caused by the LH. **Ovulation** is the production and release of an egg in each cycle. When one of the eggs first reaches maturity in the ovary, it bursts out of the follicle. The egg will live 12 to 48 hours if not fertilized. LH also causes the empty follicle to develop into a different structure that is yellow in color, called the **corpus luteum** (a Latin word meaning "yellow body"). The corpus luteum secretes some estrogen but also large amounts of **progesterone**, which has two functions:

• It further enriches and thickens the lining of the uterus.
• It causes the pituitary to decrease its production of FSH and LH to prevent more eggs from being released until progesterone levels decrease once again.

Female Reproductive Anatomy, ovulation (front view)

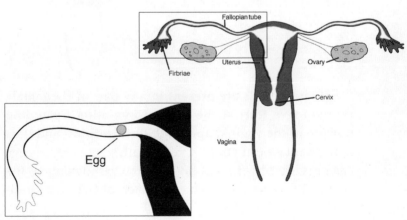

3. *The Post-ovulatory Phase* This phase begins the day after ovulation and ends the day before the reoccurence of bleeding. When conception does not occur, the corpus luteum stops functioning approximately 12 to 16 days after ovulation. The progesterone levels then decrease, which results in the shedding of the extra endometrium, or lining, in the uterus, as it is no longer needed. This shedding is called **menstruation**, or the periodic discharge of blood, mucus and tissue comprising the endometrium of the uterus. With the marked decrease in the level of progesterone, the pituitary gland will increase its production of FSH and the cycle begins again.

Female Reproductive Anatomy, post-ovulatory phase (front view)

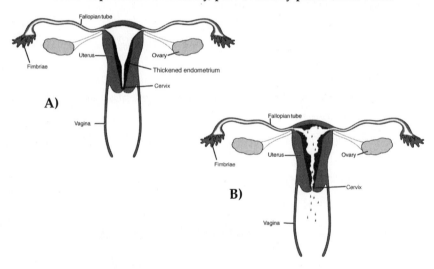

If sperm cells are present in any part of the female reproductive tract at the time of ovulation (including outside of the vaginal opening), fertilization—and thus a pregnancy—can result. Occasionally, one or more eggs can be released within 24 hours of the first ovulation. If a sperm cell penetrates each egg, fraternal twins or multiple births will most likely result.

Female Infertility

Female infertility is defined by the medical profession as the failure to become pregnant after a year of unprotected sexual intercourse. There are four basic causes of infertility: impairment of egg production and release, blocked ducts and channels, problems with implantation and age.

Impaired Egg Production and Release

Certain factors prevent or impair the production, maturation and release of the eggs. The process of ovulation is the result of the secretion and linked association of several hormones. A disturbance in just one of the hormones can result in a disruption of the process. The possible causes of the disturbance are many.

1. *Illness and Disease* Diabetes, thyroid problems, underactive adrenal glands, and diseases of the pituitary gland can negatively influence hormonal secretion.

2. *Body Weight* Excessive or insufficient body weight can be the cause of infertility. An increase in fatty tissues disrupts body hormonal balances by stimulating the production of estrogen. Conversely, if the woman is too thin, as in females who are anorexic or take part in heavy-duty physical training, there is not enough fat to promote ovulation.

3. *Environmental Factors* Illness from stress, and activities such as excessive dieting, smoking (the more a woman smokes, the less likely she is to conceive), increased alcohol consumption and exposure to radiation can also interfere with ovulation. Even caffeine consumption of over two cups per day has been linked to infertility.

4. Polycystic Ovary Syndrome (PCOS) A hormonal and metabolic condition, PCOS is the leading cause of infertility, affecting one in ten women in the United States. Increased levels of male hormones can cause erratic periods, acne, hirsutism (excessive hair on the body and face) and/or baldness at the crown of the head. Sixty percent of women with PCOS are overweight. The symptoms can be caused by other disorders and not all cases look alike. Thus, PCOS is not always easy to diagnose.

Blockages of Ducts and Channels
The blockage of ducts and channels, or structural irregularities can prevent the egg from being pulled into the fallopian tubes and proceeding toward the uterus. Likewise, sperm may be prevented from traveling up through the uterus into the tubes to meet the egg. There are several causes of this condition.

1. Problems with Cervical Mucus The cervix produces mucus to keep sperm alive and to help them move through to the uterus. Infection or hormonal abnormalities can cause the production of mucus that is insufficient in quantity to help the sperm through, or is so thick that it blocks the sperm completely from entering the uterus, or it even kills sperm.

2. Endometriosis The abnormal growth of the uterine lining outside of the uterus is called **endometriosis**. It can produce scar tissue and adhesions. Usually only moderate to severe cases cause infertility, due to damage to the ovarian tissue and fallopian tubes. Fortunately, the condition can be treated with drugs and surgery.

3. Fibroids In the uterus, **fibroids** are growths on the walls that usually do not interfere with conception. However, in some cases, they might block the fallopian tubes to prevent the sperm from reaching the egg.

4. *Disease* Pelvic inflammatory disease (PID) also can cause an obstruction of the passageway in the tubes. Sexually transmitted diseases (i.e., gonorrhea) can do the same by causing scarring of tissue and tube blockage.

5. *DES* A woman exposed to the drug DES (diethyl-stilbestrol) while she was in her mother's womb may face problems with her uterus, cervix or vagina, causing infertility.

Problems with Implantation
Certain conditions prevent the fertilized egg from implanting or growing successfully in the uterus.

1. *Low Progesterone Levels* A decrease in the level of progesterone may mean that the woman ovulates but the fertilized egg cannot implant on the wall of the uterus.

2. *Fibroids* Uterine fibroids might disturb the lining of the uterus, preventing implantation of a fertilized egg.

3. *Incompetent Cervix* If the cervix is lax or incompetent, it dilates before it should, resulting in the loss of the pregnancy in the second or third trimester, or in premature labor and delivery.

4. *Sexually Transmitted Diseases (STDs)* STDs such as chlamydia, which progress into the cervix and uterus, can cause infertility and early miscarriage.

Age

Age is a factor in infertility. Female fertility reaches its peak in the mid-twenties and then begins to decline, becoming more rapid after the age of 30. Thus, the older a woman is, the more difficulty she may experience in conceiving.

Other Reasons

Some causes of female infertility are difficult to determine, often stemming from poor health. Diseases such as renal failure and untreated diabetes can all contribute to female infertility.

As with male fertility, the optimum conditions for female fertility may sound very complicated and almost impossible to achieve. But most women are fertile and can plan their families quite easily. When we understand the wonderful workings of the male and female bodies, we certainly can appreciate the miracle of reproduction.

Chapter 5
Making a Baby: Heredity and the Process of Fertilization, Pregnancy and Birth

Thus far, you have learned about the different sex chromosomes: the X and Y, or the female and the male. These and your other 44 chromosomes play an important role in human reproduction. Heredity—how characteristics are passed from parent to offspring through genes— plays a major role in reproduction. In choosing the sex of your baby, you are choosing only one of many characteristics that your child will have. Whether the baby has blue eyes, curly hair, dimples or a pudgy nose are things you have no control over. What you do know is that your child is going to inherit special and distinct characteristics from either you or your mate. Learning the rudiments of genetics will help you understand not only how the sex of a baby is determined, but the role that heredity plays in preventing sex-linked diseases from being passed on to your children.

Likewise, choosing the sex of your baby will involve coordinating the movements of the sperm and the egg through the female's reproductive tract. The following overview of genetics and the reproductive process will help you apply this sex-selection method as you look forward to fertilization, pregnancy and birth.

Heredity

All living things, humans, animals and plants, pass on traits from one generation to another, sometimes seemingly even skipping a generation: eye color, curly or straight hair, light or dark skin, body type, height. These and other characteristics are traits determined by human genes. A human gene is a segment of a **DNA** (deoxyribonucleic acid) molecule. Everyone's body contains genetic information in their DNA, unique only to them, like their fingerprints.

Inside the nucleus of each cell are **chromosomes**, rod-shaped bodies composed of hundreds of genes arranged in a line. This genetic material is really a set of instructions for producing new cells with the same characteristics as the original, or parent, cell. Every living thing has a certain number of chromosomes. In a human being, all body cells, except for the egg and the sperm, contain 46 chromosomes, or two sets of 23 chromosomes. The two sets look very much alike. Each chromosome in one set can be paired with a particular chromosome in the other set.

When a cell begins to divide into two cells, each chromosome in the cell duplicates itself. The entire process is called **mitosis**. The duplicated chromosomes lie alongside each other in pairs. As the cell splits and separates, the pairs of chromosomes split, going in opposite directions. Thus, the two new cells that have been made have exactly the same number of identical chromosomes as the parent cell. As a result, every cell in the human body, except for the egg or sperm cell, has the identical group of chromosomes.

Why do the reproductive cells contain only half the number of chromosomes found in the rest of the cells in the body? They are formed in a special way to end up with only 23, so that when the egg and sperm unite, the fertilized egg has the 46 chromosomes of the human body—half of the chromosomes come from the mother, half from the father. The fertilized egg is now one complete cell that can replicate and divide.

Whether the fertilized egg becomes a boy or a girl is

determined by the sex chromosomes, of which there are two types. In girls, the two sex chromosomes look exactly alike and are shaped like an X. In a boy, the two chromosomes do not look alike: one is shaped like an X while the other is shorter and does not match with its partner, and is shaped more like a Y. Each sex cell contains one sex-chromosome: each egg contains one X chromosome, but a sperm cell carries either an X or a Y. If the egg is fertilized by a sperm cell with an X chromosome, then there will be two Xs (XX). In this case a girl will develop. If the sperm cell contains a Y chromosome, then the combination will be XY, and a boy will develop.

Every new body, then, inherits two genes of every trait, one from the mother and one from the father. In many traits, one gene completely overpowers the other. It is called the **dominant gene**. The less powerful one is the **recessive gene**. For instance, you have probably seen a dark-haired father and a red-haired mother who have a child who has dark hair. And you may have noticed that this same couple has another child with red hair. However, two red-haired parents will never produce a dark-haired child.

Let's look at the first couple and their dark-haired child. Since the child's hair is dark, it means that the gene for dark hair is dominant over the gene for red hair. Each one of that child's cells would contain a gene for red hair (**r**) and a gene for dark hair (**D**). Because there are two chromosomes paired together, one from the mom and one from the dad, they are shown as a pair. The paired genes would be written as **Dr**. The father has received his two genes from his parents. Thus, his trait of dark hair could be shown in two ways: **DD**, meaning that a dark hair gene came from each of his parents, or **Dr** if, perhaps, his mother had dark hair but his father had red hair. Now, when considering the mother of the dark-haired child, because red hair is a recessive trait, the mother's pairing would show as **rr**. Each parent would only give one of the genes in the pair. The possible traits that might be seen in their offspring can be shown by means of a table called a Punnett's Square.

Father has dark hair (DD), Mother has red hair (rr)
(D=dark hair r=red hair)

Father DD Mother rr	D	D
r	Dr	Dr
r	Dr	Dr

In this example, all the children would have the dark hair of their father because they would all have a dominant (**D**) dark hair gene (a 100 percent chance of having dark hair).

Father has dark hair (Dr), Mother has red hair (rr)
(D=dark hair r=red hair)

Heredity,
Fertilization,
Pregnancy and
Birth

Father Dr / Mother rr	D	r
r	Dr	rr
r	Dr	rr

In the second example, two of the children might have dark hair. Two might be redheads like their mother. To say it another way, there is a 50 percent chance that the child will have dark hair and a 50 percent chance that the child will be a redhead.

Disease and Sex-linked Genes

But dominant and recessive genes can have more serious implications than hair texture or eye color. If there is a negative characteristic on a recessive gene, the domninant gene will overrule, or overpower, this weaker gene so the negative trait does not manifest itself. Only when the two recessive genes are together will the characteristic be revealed. Negative characteristics include genes for diseases or other disorders, such as cystic fibrosis. Cystic fibrosis is an inherited childhood disease characterized by the failure of the glands that secrete mucus and digestive enzymes. The disease involves the lungs, liver, pancreas and other organs and a child with cystic fibrosis is very susceptible to infections. This disease will manifest itself in the child much like the trait for red hair will: one or both parents carry one gene for cystic fibrosis that is paired with a dominant gene that overpowers it, canceling out the disease. Therefore, neither of the child's parents is known to have the disease because they have no signs or symptoms. The parents are said to be **carriers** of the disease. Unfortunately, when each of the carrier parents contributes that one recessive gene, the recessive trait is displayed and the child has cystic fibrosis.

Often, these negative characteristics are located on sex-linked genes: genes carried on the sex-determining X or Y chromosomes. This means that they are diseases or conditions that will manifest in only one sex. Some sex-linked genes on the X chromosome can cause harmful effects such as color blindness, hemophilia and Duchenne's muscular dystrophy. These conditions always occur in males because males have only one X chromosome. The other Y chromosome has no dominant power to stop the occurrence of the condition. The lucky females, however, have two X chromosomes. Thus, if one X has the recessive "bad" condition, the other X may have the dominant "good" gene and so the symptoms of the condition (e.g., color blindness, abnormal bleeding) will not show, although she will be a carrier of the recessive gene and may pass it on to her children.

The Y chromosome, being smaller than the X, carries fewer genes. It seems that the only trait known so far to be carried on the Y chromosome is hairy ears, which only males will display because only males have a Y chromosome.

It can be interesting to look at yourself, your parents, your mate and your children to see what dominant or recessive traits everyone has, and, therefore, which child is more like which parent or which is a real "mixed bag".

Fertilization

Fertilization means the union of the male and female sex cells to produce a one-celled individual called a zygote. This can happen as a result of two things. Either

- the tip of the penis comes in contact with the outside of the woman's body near the opening of her vagina (before or after ejaculation), and some sperm finds its way in and up through her uterus to the egg; or
- during sexual intercourse, the male ejaculates between 200 million to 600 million sperm into the vagina and the sperm swim up through the cervix and uterus into the fallopian tubes and one penetrates the released egg.

Fertilization

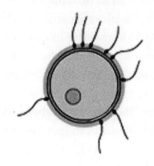

Fewer than 100 sperm are in the tubes when the egg and sperm join. As soon as the head and neck of one sperm enter the egg, the tail drops off and all remaining sperm are denied entry. Only one sperm can unite with the egg. The sperm head then forms itself into a special structure called the **nucleus**, and moves towards the nucleus of the egg. Amazingly, as it does this, all the other sperm outside whip their tails at precisely the same time and rhythm to cause a rippling effect which rotates the egg clockwise, with increasing speed, propelling the egg down the fallopian tube. Inside, the sperm nucleus joins with the nucleus of the egg. At that precise moment, a new single-celled individual, or **zygote**, has been conceived.

The zygote continues down the tube, on its journey, and, approximately 24 to 36 hours after fertilization, begins mitosis, and thus starts to divide into two cells, identical to each other, then four cells and eight cells. Each cell division takes about 15 hours. After about three days the zygote is made up of eight cells, each capable of developing into a complete human being. (This is the way identical twins are made. Sometimes the embryo splits spontaneously, resulting in two genetically identical beings of the same sex.)

When the cell division proceeds normally, in the next three days the eight cells become 16, then 32, and so on, resulting in the formation of what one would describe as a ball of cells called a **blastocyst**. The cells are all around the outside of the ball and the inside is filled with fluid. The size of the blastocyst is still the same size as the original egg because each new cell divides into two smaller cells and they all become packed into the same area. The blastocyst reaches the uterus, where it floats around. After about a week, it starts to increase in size and attaches itself to the thickened wall of the uterus. This is called implantation and the blastocyst can also be called an **embryo**. Implantation generally occurs about 7 to 14 days after fertilization of the egg. At this point, pregnancy begins.

Implantation

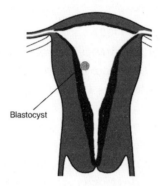

Blastocyst

Pregnancy

When the embryo is in the blastocyst stage, the cells are very similar to each other. In about another week, though, the cells start to differentiate, or become specialized, in order to perform the different functions of the various tissues and organs in the body. An organ of tissue and blood vessels, called the **placenta**, develops around the embryo in the uterus. At the same time, a membranous sac containing fluid develops around the embryo to protect it. The sac is called the **amniotic sac** and the fluid is termed **amniotic fluid**.

The placenta has two functions. It transfers nutrients and oxygen into the embryo's blood system from the mother, and takes back waste products from the embryo. The embryo is connected to the placenta by the umbilical cord. The placenta also takes over for the corpus luteum and maintains high levels of progesterone, necessary to sustain the pregnancy.

The amount of time from conception to birth, or the gestation period, for a human being is approximately 38 to 40 weeks. This period can be divided into three blocks of time, or **trimesters**, each about three months in duration. Major developmental changes occur within each trimester.

First Trimester (weeks 1–12)
One of the signs of pregnancy is the missed menstrual period. Naturally, no bleeding has occurred because the rich lining of the uterus is needed for the developing embryo.

By the time the embryo is four weeks old it is 45 millimeters/less than one quarter of an inch long. There is a heart that circulates blood through its vessels. The brain is another organ that develops early on. No eyes, nose or ears are yet to be seen. Small buds, which will be arms and legs, are showing and the digestive system is beginning to form. The embryo even has a tail! Proper nutrition and abstinence from alcohol, smoking and drugs are vitally important in the early weeks of the pregnancy, often before some women even realize they are pregnant.

By eight weeks, the embryo is 2.5 centimeters/1 inch long and weighs almost 1 gram. The head is large compared to the body. Its face and features are forming. It has eyes covered with eyelids (which remain shut until week 24) and organs are formed but not developed, except for the stomach and kidneys, which have begun to function. Arms and legs are beginning to show and the tail is disappearing. At eight to nine weeks, the embryo begins to form its first bone cells. Once this happens, the embryo is now called a **fetus**.

By the end of 12 weeks, all the major organs have begun their development. The fetus is 9 centimeters/3.5

inches long and it can now swallow. Nerve and muscle coordination is improving. The sex of the fetus can be identified using ultrasound technology.

As mentioned, the developing fetus receives all its nutrients and oxygen from the mother by way of the placenta and umbilical cord. But it may receive harmful substances also. Whatever the mother eats, drinks or inhales will go into the fetus. Some substances can permanently damage the developing fetus. Cigarette smoke causes the fetus's blood vessels to constrict or to close and become narrower. This can prevent enough oxygen from getting to those vital developing tissues. Alcohol may affect the brain, central nervous system and other physical developments. The liver of an adult helps to get rid of harmful substances in the body; however, the fetus's liver is not even able to help out when it is at full term or ready to be born. Even a newborn's liver is still immature.

Certain drugs may cause deformities in the developing fetus. For example, thalidomide, a drug prescribed in the 1950s to help reduce the mother's nausea in the first trimester, interferred with the proper development of the fetus' arms and legs. Many babies were born with missing or severely deformed limbs. (Thalidomide use was discontinued in 1961.) For this reason, no drugs of any kind (even medication for a headache or for a cold) should be taken without the direction of a physician. Proper nutrition and health habits in this first trimester are critically important to the developing fetus. These habits should also continue right through the pregnancy in order to prevent deformity, miscarriage and low birth weight.

Second Trimester (weeks 12–24)
At 16 weeks, the placenta is too small to surround the fetus, so it moves to one side. The skeleton begins to

form, the brain grows rapidly and the nervous system begins to function.

By 20 weeks, the fetus is clearly human in appearance. It is 25 centimeters/10 inches long and weighs about 300 grams/11 ounces. It has some hair! As the fetus moves its new muscles and flexes, the mother begins to feel movement.

At the end of 24 weeks, the fetus is 32 centimeters/13 inches long and weighs about 650 grams/1 pound, 7 ounces. The eyelids have separated but a thin membrane covers the pupils. Most organs are formed but are not fully developed or mature enough for the fetus to live outside the mother's body. The fetus's movements become increasingly vigorous.

Third Trimester (weeks 24–38)

The skin of the fetus is wrinkled now but fat deposits begin to build up. During this last trimester, the fetus grows rapidly in size, and begins to move around within the amniotic sac, kicking and stretching. The immune system develops around this time. Proper nutrition is still very important, especially to aid in the building up of vital brain tissue. If the mother does not properly nourish herself and the fetus, the nutrients in the mother's body will be used for the fetus, possibly causing permanent health problems in some women.

By the end of the eighth month, the fetus is about 46 centimeters/18 inches long and weighs about 2.5 kilograms/5 pounds. Fat has been deposited beneath the skin and the fetus has a 90 percent chance of surviving if born now.

At full term, when it is ready to be born, the fetus is approximately 50 centimeters/20 inches and weighs about 3 kilograms/7 pounds, 4 ounces. Often boys weigh about 100 grams/4 ounces more than girls.

Birth

The whole process of giving birth is called **labor**. Although it seems to be a mystery as to what triggers the process or says, "Okay, the baby is ready to be born", it is known that there are sudden and dramatic changes in hormone levels that start the process. There is a sharp drop in the levels of progesterone and estrogen, which have been sustaining the pregnancy. At the same time, the pituitary gland in the mother produces another hormone, oxytocin, which stimulates the uterus to contract and open the birth canal. Labor is divided into three stages, dilation, expulsion and the placental stage. It's all so amazing, isn't it?

Dilation
The first stage is the longest and begins with the first signs that labor is starting. The woman may experience one or more of some of the typical signs listed below.

- A mucus "plug"or a bloody, mucous discharge from the vagina may be noticed.
- The amniotic sac may break and the water inside may be expelled. (The woman may initially think she has been incontinent or had an "accident" as her water breaks.)
- The woman may experience tightening around her belly, lower back pain, menstrual-like pains or a combination of all three.

During this stage, the cervix to thins and then opens, or dilates, to allow for the baby's head to pass through. The contractions become harder and more intense as this stage progresses.

Expulsion

In the second stage, the contractions of the uterus become so forceful and strong that the baby is pushed through the cervix into the vagina or birth canal. The vagina will shorten and the baby's head will appear at the vaginal opening. The head is usually facing down after it comes through the opening, but then the baby rotates, or turns and faces sideways to make it easier for the shoulders and rest of the body to pass through.

Most babies are born head first. If any other part of the baby's body starts to come out first, it is called a **breech birth**. If the baby cannot be turned around, or if there are any complications in the mother or baby, the doctor will make a small cut through the woman's abdomen and into the uterus and take the baby out. This is called a **Caesarean section (C-section)**.

Placental Stage

After the baby is born (either vaginally or by C-section), the placenta comes off the wall of the uterus and, with the umbilical cord, is expelled or removed. This usually happens within 10 to 30 minutes after the baby is born. The expelled placenta is also called the **afterbirth**.

Part Three

The Method: Determining Ovulation and Timing Intercourse

Now that all of the background information has been covered, we are ready to get into the method. Choosing the sex of your baby is dependent on determining the time of the woman's ovulation so that intercourse can occur at exactly the right time, either a few days before ovulation to increase the chances of having a girl or at the time of ovulation to increase the chances of having a boy. But first, how can you know when ovulation occurs?

The key to determining ovulation and the time you are most fertile is noting the body's changes and understanding what these physical signs mean. Chapter 6 discusses ovulation and its primary and secondary signs, including changes in the cervical mucus (CM), the cervix and the body's basal temperature (BBT) as well as hormonal testing. Chapter 7 shows you how to chart your menstrual cycle, noting the signs that indicate when you are fertile, and Chapter 8 teaches you how to interpret your chart to determine the exact time of ovulation. Finally, Chapter 9 explains in detail how to time intercourse for the desired sex and reviews some other factors that can increase your chances of success.

Chapter 6
Reading the Signs of Female Fertility

It is important to be able to read the signs of female fertility in order to successfully plan and prevent pregnancies. Each of these signs is found by observing the progression menstrual cycle. The following is a discussion of the menstrual cycle and ovulation, the primary and secondary signs of fertilty and the importance of understanding fertility to prevent unwanted pregnancies.

Three Phases of Ovulation

The menstrual cycle is divided into three phases.

1. Pre-ovulatory phase (includes menstruation)
2. Ovulation
3. Post-ovulatory phase

Menstruation

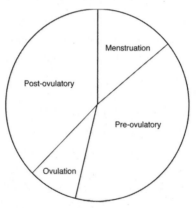

During each of these phases, the hormones released by the ovaries, estrogen and progesterone, cause signs that can be recognized and interpreted to determine which phase of the menstrual cycle a woman is in.

The Pre-ovulatory Phase

The pre-ovulatory, or estrogenic, phase begins the first day of menstruation and ends at the time of ovulation. During this phase, the lining of the uterus is being shed as the woman has her period. The pituitary gland has released the follical stimulating hormone (FSH), stimulating the follicles in the ovaries to mature. The developing follicle secretes estrogen into the bloodstream. This hormone causes the cervical crypts to produce mucus. This mucus is observable in the vaginal area and creates a change in sensation, from feeling dry to feeling wet and slippery as ovulation approaches. At the same time, the cervix is low, tilted, firm and closed and the basal body temperature (the temperature of the body at rest) is generally low. A peak amount of estrogen is also needed to cause the maturation and release of the egg. The length of the pre-ovulatory phase is determined by the time needed to cause hormonal stimulation that will ripen the egg. Thus, the duration of this phase could be minimal, such as six days, or lengthy, such as 60 days. There is nothing wrong with either length. The nature of the signs of this phase may vary from cycle to cycle, and from woman to woman.

Ovulation

Ovulation is the release of the egg from the ovary. Sometimes ovulation is delayed or does not occur (this is called a **monophasic** or **anovulatory**, cycle). There are many factors influencing the exact timing of ovulation. These factors are related to circumstances of the pre-ovulatory phase that influence the amount of estrogen released. For example, stress, disease and premenopause, among other factors, can all cause changes in hormone levels. Should ovulation not occur, the pituitary gland continues to stimulate the follicles in the ovaries and the cervical crypts will still produce mucus. The changes the woman notices in her mucus may make it seem as if the ovaries were "trying hard" to ovulate (the mucus alternates between characteristics which appear to be almost fertile and those which are infertile). For example, a woman may notice these types of changes during breast-feeding.

At ovulation, usually only one egg is released. As previously mentioned, occasionally a second egg (or more) will be released, usually within 12 hours of the first. Once the ovulation phase is over, no other egg will be released during that cycle (i.e., until the next cycle has begun). The cervical mucus at this stage is abundant and slippery; the cervix is high, straight, open and soft; and the basal body temperature rises.

Post-ovulatory Phase

The post-ovulatory phase begins after ovulation and continues until the first day of the next menstrual cycle. After ovulation, the ovarian follicles continue to secret estrogen. At the same time, the corpus luteum secretes progesterone, which helps to maintain the lining of the uterus so it is ready for a fertilized egg. Progesterone also changes the characteristics of the mucus produced by the crypts, making it pasty, sticky or dry, and it keeps the basal body temperature high or raises it. In this phase, the cervix returns to a low, tilted, firm and closed position.

The post-ovulatory phase is consistent in length for every woman. Once ovulation occurs, a woman will get her period 12 to 16 days (note the 14-day average) later, unless she conceives. While a woman may get her period 12 days after ovulation in one cycle, and then 15 days after ovulation in the next cycle, she knows her period will always come she knows her period will always come somewhere between 12 and 16 days after ovulation. Although the pre-ovulatory phase can vary in length from woman to woman, this post-ovulatory interval is true for every woman, every cycle. To illustrate this point, I have examples of the cycles of three different women. Note that the time period after ovulation (Ov), the post-ovulatory phase, is almost the same length, varying between 12 and 16 days.

Pre-ovulatory Days (8)	Ov	Post-ovulatory Days (12 days)
1 2 3 4 5 6 7 8	9	10 11 12 13 14 15 16 17 18 19 20 21

Pre-ovulatory Days (14)	Ov	Post-ovulatory Days (16 days)
1 2 3 4 5 6 7 8 9 10 11 12 13 14	15	16 17 18 19 20 21 22 23 24 25 26 27 28 29 30 31

Pre-ovulatory Days (46)	Ov	Post-ovulatory Days (14 days)
1 2 3 4 5 6 7 8 9 10...... 40 41 42 43 44 45 46	47	48 49 50 51 52 53 54 55 56 57 58 59 60 61

I had cycles similar to the third one. Understanding my fertility was beneficial not only for determining when to begin or prevent a pregnancy but also for ensuring a secure feeling in knowing when my period would be coming.

Primary Signs of Female Fertility

Amazingly, when a woman becomes attuned to her body's signs, she will be able to pinpoint the day she ovulates by noting the sometimes slight changes in the way she feels mentally and physically and by observing one or more of the three major natural fertility signs: the cervical mucus (CM), the changes in the position of the cervix and her basal body temperature (BBT).

Cervical Mucus (CM)
It is astonishing to realize that the woman's body displays signals indicating what is happening inside, yet

most women don't realize what these signs mean. A little knowledge is truly valuable.

The majority of females experience a small discharge from the vagina that they might notice in their underpants: sometimes, there will be a yellow, dry, flaky substance on them; at other times, there is a thick, clumpy discharge. As you saw in the overview above, both are telling a story about what is happening in your cycle, and you must pay attention to each.

The glands in the cervix produce a healthy and normal discharge, termed **cervical mucus**. It can be either **infertile** or **fertile mucus**. Normally the sperm will die very quickly once inside the woman, usually within 12 to 24 hours, but fertile mucus envelops the sperm cells so that they may live for up to six days inside the female reproductive tract. This mucus also nourishes the sperm cells by providing energy requirements and may possibly help the sperm fertilize the egg.

There are three different types of mucus produced by the cervix. A woman may notice one or more of them as her period ends, depending on the length of her cycle.

1. Infertile G-type Mucus This mucus is the first type *produced as menstruation is ceasing or after it has finished*. In a short cycle, this mucus may not be noticed. Infertile G-type mucus is a pasty, infertile barrier mucus that is opaque and can be sticky or crumbly. It forms an impenetrable barrier to sperm. The mucus sometimes resembles old-fashioned library paste, looking whitish-yellow on the underpants. If you scratch the mucus, it will flake off. Due to a lack of moisture in G-type mucus, the vaginal area can feel dry or sticky. The woman may not experience the same amount of lubrication, or vaginal wetness, during intercourse that she does on other days of her cycle.

2. Infertile L-type Mucus The second type of infertile mucus is L-type mucus, characterized by "beads" of mucus that cause a thick, clumpy texture. It is a sign of *beginning fertility*. The job of this mucus is to make the vagina less acidic, so that sperm can live in it; it is also intended to form a slight barrier, trapping defective sperm. This type of mucus can cause a wet feeling around the opening of the vagina and appears creamy and bead-like. If you put some mucus between your thumb and index finger, you will notice that as you pull your fingers apart, it may start to stretch but will break.

3. Fertile S-type Mucus Also termed fertile mucus, S-type mucus is indicative of the *fertile phase* of the cycle, or the period of time during which intercourse is likely to cause fertilization of the egg. Its appearence helps pinpoint the **Peak day**. This fertile mucus has the appearance and texture of raw egg white, being clearer than the L-type. S-type mucus is also called spinnbarkeit (a German word for spiderweb). It is very stretchy, making strings or loops that can look like strands of a web. It is essential for conception, causing watery channels in which the sperm can be carried. The sperm may go right up into the uterus or be kept for a while in the specialized folds of the cervix where S-type mucus is produced. When observed under an electron microscope, the mucus appears to be like a bundle of little fibres, with small spaces between them, making "canals". The sperm are rereleased on contact with fluid from the uterus, enabling the life of the sperm to be prolonged. The woman will probably feel wet around the opening of the vagina. There can be an increase in wet mucus in her underpants and sometimes a woman may think S-type mucus is a sign of a vaginal infection, but it isn't. Alcohol and drugs can alter this pattern, sometimes causing a decrease in mucus production, making the observation of these signs difficult.

Observation of the mucus and distinguishing between the three types is essential for determining if you are in a fertile or infertile phase of your cycle. However, the *sensation* of mucus is also a very important sign. Sometimes, very close to ovulation, the mucus can be so fluid that observing it is difficult. However, there may be a feeling or sensation of wetnes, or lubrication, at the vaginal opening. For some women, the mucus can be pink-tinged. Spotting (light, non-menstrual bleeding caused by a change in hormone levels), or even heavier non-menstrual bleeding may mask mucus signs. Thus, a woman may be more aware that she is ovulating by her sensations than by actual observations. In addition, some woman may feel a pain on either side of the lower abdomen, called mittelschmerz. The pain can be dull, diffuse or even sharp, lasting a few minutes to a few hours.

G-type mucus can appear in both the pre- and post-ovulatory phases, while L-type mucus appears in the pre-ovulatory phase closer to ovulation. S-type mucus will only appear in the few days before and after ovulation, during a woman's fertile phase.

The Peak Day and After   The last day the mucus presents one or more of the primary signs of fertile S-type mucus by appearance and/or sensation is termed the **Peak day**. The estrogen level is at its highest on this day. The peak mucus signal occurs, on average, 14 hours before ovulation. In about 85 percent of women, the peak signal occurs within 24 hours of ovulation; in 95 percent of women, it occurs within 48 hours ovulation. Because the egg can live for 12 to 24 hours, **the fertile phase lasts for**

three days after the Peak day. The Peak day is important because it allows you to determine the bracket of time when you are fertile. Having this time frame allows you to time intercourse closer to ovulation for a boy and right at the beginning of your fertile period for a girl.

After ovulation, the progesterone level rises. Secreted by the corpus luteum, progesterone changes the characteristics of the mucus so that it does not have the stretchy, raw egg-white appearance. The wet feeling outside the vagina disappears; the mucus becomes pasty, sticky, or is gone. While some women will have a pasty mucus until their next period, others will notice no discharge and have a constant dry feeling outside the vagina for the remainder of the cycle. For others, there may be wet mucus and a wet sensation a few days prior to their period, but this mucus is not fertile, it is just part of the normal change for those particular individuals.

Irregularities in Mucus   Certain drugs can affect the mucus pattern. Some tranquilizers, for example, chlorpromazine, may cause a delay in ovulation. Cytotoxic (cell-killing) drugs used in cancer treatment can prevent mucus production by their direct action on the ovaries. When using antibiotics, a woman may notice a change in her mucus pattern, although it may be caused more by the stress of the illness that is being treated than by the side-effects of the medication. Women on antibiotics for a chronic illness can learn to interpret their CM pattern successfully. Other drugs that may affect the production of mucus are hormones (especially progesterone and estrogen) and antihistamines.

Cervical mucus is the main fertility sign altering a woman that ovulation is approaching and confirming that it has occurred. Reading the signs of CM is the most reliable way of knowing when ovulation is approaching and, therefore, preventing or planning a pregnancy. Many people have used these observations as a means of natural family planning, known to some as the Billings method.

Changes in the Cervix

Throughout the cycle, the cervix changes texture and position as the uterus rises. These changes help confirm the other signs of each phase of the cycle. A manual examination of the cervix will reveal these qualities.

Positions of the Cervix

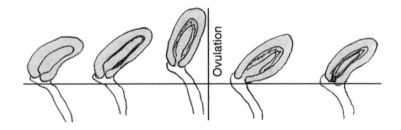

1. Cervix at Menstruation The cervix is low, tilted, firm and closed. It feels similar to a dimple if the woman has never delivered a baby vaginally, or if there has been a vaginal birth, it will feel irregularly-shaped.

2. Cervix at Ovulation The cervix rises, straightens and softens (the feeling is comparable to the softness of one's lips) and it is more open.

3. Cervix after Ovulation The cervix is once again closed, firm and low.

Basal Body Temperature (BBT)

When you awake in the morning (hopefully after a restful sleep), before you move and get out of bed, take your temperature. Do not use the thermometer you have for checking to see if you have a fever. It is more accurate to use a special thermometer, one that can read very small changes in temperature. This is a thermometer that measures your basal body temperature (BBT). As stated previously, your BBT is the temperature of your body at rest. It represents the minimum amount of energy needed to maintain the basic body functions when the body is resting.

Progesterone has an effect on the BBT of a woman. During her cycle, a woman's BBT will change, indicating that a different phase has been reached. As you will note in the graph below, this change is very slight; it is not in degrees, as in a fever, but in *points* of a degree.

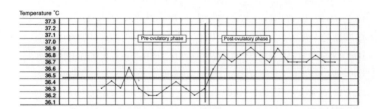

1. BBT in Pre-ovulatory Phase The pre-ovulatory phase is characterized by a low temperature (T) phase. The above graph shows that the temperature fluctuates up or down by only 0.1 or 0.2 °C/°F.

2. BBT at Ovulation Further into the cycle, approaching ovulation, progesterone causes the temperature to rise or shift 0.1 to 0.5 °C/0.2 to 0.8 °F (averaging 0.2 °C or 0.4 °F) over a period of one to four days

3. BBT in Post-ovulatory Phase In the post-ovulatory phase, the temperature remains high, reflecting the life span of the corpus luteum (12 to16 days). The temperature drops either just before or during menstruation unless conception has occurred.

Studies have been done to determine the relationship of the rise in BBT to the exact time of ovulation. One study, done in 1980, concluded that this rise occurred within two days prior to two days after ovulation. Another, done in the same year, stated that the rise occurs at ovulation or just prior to ovulation, while a report in 1982 reported that ovulation occurred prior to the BBT rise. Frequently, a drop in the temperature is seen just before the rise.

Irregularities in BBT Most of the research seems to agree that ovulation usually takes place the day before the temperature rise (one reported a half of a day prior to the rise). When the temperature stays high for three days, it indicates that the egg has been released. Unfortunately, there can be false rises due to factors such as changes in climate, disturbed sleeps, fatigue, a late night out, emotional trauma or excessive use of alcohol. While no research has shown that the taking of tranquilizers, sleeping pills or antibiotics have a direct effect, the reasons for taking the medications might influence the BBT.

Secondary Signs of Female Fertility

Around the time of ovulation, some women (about 15 to 25 percent) will describe a pain that they feel in their abdomen or lower back. Medically, the pain is called, mittelschmerz, meaning the pain that comes in the middle of the cycle (assuming a regular 28-day cycle). In about 91 percent of the women who experience it, the pain comes 24 to 48 hours before ovulation. For some, there is a dull ache that may even last a couple of days. A rush of blood that goes to the follicle and forms a type of clot may be the cause of this dull pain. For others, there may be a sharp pain or stabbing feeling that can be either very short in length, or last a couple of hours. In some women, the pain is almost incapacitating and medication is needed to offset the discomfort. The more intense pain may be caused by the egg's bursting out of the follicle. Finally, other women may experience a combination of these two sensations, or, perhaps, other sensations that seem to be unique to them, which help them pinpoint ovulation.

As ovulation approaches, some women may also see or feel other secondary signs.

- The oil-producing glands secrete less oil. The complexion may be clearer.
- There may be fluid retention causing breast tenderness, a bloated feeling and/or irritability.
- The energy level may rise.
- Spotting, or light, non-menstrual bleeding from the vagina, may occur.

Other Indicators of Female Fertility

There are two other ways that a woman is able to determine the time of ovulation: both involve testing hormone levels in the body. Please note that these methods can be costly, and I do not recommend using them alone. However, they are good supplementary measures when used with the observation of the primary and secondary signs of fertility outlined above.

Ovulation Kits

Some couples like to use a kit to help them to understand or to confirm what the woman's signs are telling them as to when ovulation is occurring. While I have not used an ovulation kit, I know of several women who have in order to validate their observations. The test done by the ovulation kit measures the amount of luteinizing hormone (LH) present in the urine. Just before ovulation, there is a surge in LH. When testing, the first positive occurs between 16 and 28 hours before ovulation.

Some prescription drugs, such as Pergonal, Cyclomen and Clomid may affect the results. It is important to consult with your physician or pharmacist about how any medications will affect ovulation-test results. Certain rare medical conditions and the onset of menopause may cause elevated levels of LH. Also, should a woman not ovulate during any one of her cycles, she will not see any LH surge.

Blood Tests

Blood tests can also be done to measure the level of hormones that fluctuate at different times in the cycle. These tests require a visit to the doctor and can be a costly option.

Preventing Unwanted Pregnancy

As suggested earlier, being familiar with the signs of fertility is important for both planning and preventing pregnancies. Because sperm can survive in the female reproductive tract for a number of days, it is possible to become pregnant not only at the time of ovulation, but several days before or after, during your fertile phase. The time when a woman ovulates is unique to her; for example, some women have found that they ovulate during their periods. For this reason it is important to pay close attention to your own cycle and to use a form of birth control, preferably a condom, without disrupting your cycle. I will be discussing the role of birth control throughout the following chapters.

Chapter 7
Charting Your Cycle

To be able to fully understand your own menstrual cycle, you must keep a record of the primary and secondary signs of fertility that you experience. I will discuss how to chart and interpret the characteristics of the cervical mucus (CM), the cervical changes and the basal body temperature (BBT), as well as the secondary signs of fertility, as described in the last chapter. An example of this chart can found in Appendix C for you to copy or enlarge for your own use.

But before you begin charting, it is important to note a few factors which may interfere with how you read and record the various signs and symptoms of fertility.

1. Sexual Intercourse and Charting Your Cycle When you are first learning to recognize the different types of cervical mucus and your cycle's pattern, it is necessary to abstain from intercourse. The seminal fluid and the vaginal secretions from sexual excitement may cause confusion for the woman just starting to read her CM. Once the woman becomes more proficient at interpreting her signs, making love should be limited to the end of the day. Intercourse in the morning may interfere with seeing the possible change to fertile mucus that could have occurred during the night.

2. Birth Control and Charting Your Cycle When you are comfortable enough with reading your CM, you may want to begin having sex again. Natural family planning, that is, charting and reading the woman's cycle to prevent a pregnancy, is the method of birth control a couple can use when trying to pinpoint ovulation. However, I suggest the use of a *non-lubricated* condom to prevent pregnancy and as a way to improve the accuracy of your readings of fertility signs. After unprotected intercourse the semen from the male may be confused with the natural discharge from the cervix and make reading the signs of fertility difficult. The condom prevents the semen from being deposited in the vagina and prevents muddled readings. Foam and spermicidal jellies will also confuse the signs, while the use of a diaphragm or cervical cap allows the semen into the vagina. Using a condom, however, does not interfere with the secretions or the reading of the cervical mucus.

Other artificial methods of birth control are not to be used when a woman is observing her cycle, because of the way they prevent pregnancy. For example, the purpose of the birth control pill is to prevent the woman from ovulating. With no egg released, there is nothing to fertilize, therefore, there can be no pregnancy. Obviously, she will also not display the signs of fertility. When a couple wishes to conceive, the woman should stop using the Pill and remain off it for at least three months. This way, she will have a chance to observe several cycles to determine when she ovulates. An intrauterine device (IUD) works by either preventing fertilization, or by not allowing the fertilized egg to be implanted on the wall of the uterus. Although its presence will not interfere with the reading of her fertility signs, the IUD must be removed and the woman should have a couple of natural cycles before the couple tries to conceive.

The only artificial method of birth control I recommend using is the non-lubricated condom.

3. Drugs Although research has not shown that medications change the BBT, there is a correlation between the two. For example, Aspirin, Tylenol or ibuprofin may lower the body's temperature if you are taking them to reduce a fever. Antihistamines may have the same drying effect on the mucus of the cervix as they do on the mucus of the nasal passageways. It is imporant to record any medications that you take for a temporary period of time, and why.

As you chart, you are looking to identify the three phases of your cycle: the **pre-ovulatory infertile phase**, the period before ovulation when pregnancy cannot occur; the **fertile phase**, before, during and after ovulation when pregnancy can occur; and the **post-ovulatory infertile phase**, the time when the egg has died and conception is not possible.

What follows is a breakdown of the chart and an explanation of how to record the various signs of fertility. Please note that the numbers 1 to 12 written along the right side of the sample charts in this chapter correspond with different parts of my explanation so that you may better understand how to record and interpret your chart. These numbers are also on the blank chart in Appendix C. I have also provided a series of symbols for you to record each fertility sign; the legend at the bottom of the blank chart in Appedix C will remind you what to write.

Days and Dates

You want to begin your chart on the first day of your period. Write the name of the month(s) of the cycle you are beginning to chart. Then refer to line 2 to number the days of your cycle. In the first box, mark the first day of your period as day 1. Next, refer to line 1 to record the calandar date for this cycle, beginning with the first day of your period. In the example below the woman's period began on August 26, the first day of her cycle.

Months __Aug. - Sept.__

| Day of Month | 26 | 27 | 28 | 29 | 30 | 31 | 1 | 2 | 3 | 4 | 5 | 6 | 7 | 8 | 9 | 10 | 11 | 12 | 13 | 14 | 15 | 16 | 17 | 18 | 19 | 20 | 21 | 22 | 23 | 24 | 25 | 26 | 1 |
| Day of Cycle | 1 | 2 | 3 | 4 | 5 | 6 | 7 | 8 | 9 | 10 | 11 | 12 | 13 | 14 | 15 | 16 | 17 | 18 | 19 | 20 | 21 | 22 | 23 | 24 | 25 | 26 | 27 | 28 | 29 | 30 | 31 | 32 | 2 |

Charting Cervical Mucus(CM)

When charting the cervical mucus, you are observing two things: the appearance of the mucus discharge and the vaginal sensations. Refer to lines 3 and 4 on the sample chart found on page 110.

It is important to check yourself and look in your underpants each time you go to the bathroom. You'll also find it easier to do this check after you have exercised or have had a bowel movement.

You should wait until the end of the day to record only the most fertile sign that appeared during the day. You may want to keep a diary with you during the day to write down the signs each time you check.

Mucus Appearance (line 3)
When you begin your period, you will chart a **P** for any day that there is a colored discharge. After the period ends, you will continue to check the nature and appearance of any discharge.

•*Look* It is not necessary to check inside the vaginal opening for mucus. Simply look for any mucus on *white* toilet tissue after using it to dry yourself, and observe any discharge in your underpants. Is there any mucus? What colour is the mucus—creamy, yellow, clear, opaque? Is it dry, flaky, sticky, wetter or more liquid, slippery, stretchy? Is there much of it? Does it sit in a lump?

•*Touch* Feel the mucus with your fingers. Does it feel dry, wetter (or more liquid, creamy, beadlike, et cetera) slippery, stretchy? Draw your fingers slowly apart to check the stretch.

•*Write* Use the letters and symbols I've provided, or use

your own, and record your observations on the correct day each evening. Chart a **P** for any day you have your period; **D** if the mucus is dry or there is nothing to observe; **F** for any day the mucus is flaky; **S** for any day it is sticky; **M** for any mucus that is wetter, L-type (or more liquid, creamy, beadlike, et cetera); and an **M with a circle around it** for any stretchy, slippery mucus. *Record only the most fertile sign of the day.*

Day of Cycle	1	2	3	4	5	6	7	8	9	10	11	12	13	14	15	16	17	18	19	20	21	22	23	24	25	26	27	28	29	30	31	32	2
Appearance	P	P	P	P	P	D	D	F	S	M	M	Ⓜ	Ⓜ	D	D	S	S	D	D	D	D	D	D	D	D	D	D	P					3
Sensation									D	D	D	S	W	W	W	W	S	S	S	D	D	D	D	D	D	D	D	D					4

Vaginal Sensations (line 4)
As you go about your day, be aware of your body. What does the opening of your vagina feel like? Do you feel dry (**D**), sticky (**S**) or really wet (**W**)? It is important to be aware of the sensations because the mucus may become so fluid that you will be unable to detect any. Write down the appropriate symbols to indicate the sensations at the end of the day.

Example of a Typical CM Chart
The chart above shows how a cycle generally reveals itself this way through cervical mucus.

1. Period There are days of bleeding, the duration varying from woman to woman. A **P** is charted on every day that there is a colored discharge, whether red- or brown-tinged, copious or scant (here it is days 1 to 5).

2. Basic Infertile Pattern (BIP) Next, there may be a non-changing mucus that is dry or flaky and a dry vaginal sensation. This is termed the Basic Infertile Pattern (BIP) and charted with a **D** or an **F** (here it is days 6, 7, 8). The BIP days are those where the infertile cervical mucus (most likely G-type) remains the same consistency (whether it be dry, flaky, sticky or thick) for several consecutive days.

3. *Fertile Phase* A change in the BIP indicates the start of the fertile phase and happens, on average, about six days before ovulation. The mucus is usually L-type, and is gummy, or thick and opaque. The opening of the vagina may feel sticky and the surrounding tissue may even feel soft and swollen. You can chart and **S** (sticky) for this type of mucus, and an **S** (sticky**)** or an **W** (wet) for the sensation (here it is day 9). You'll notice when the mucus starts to shift to fertile S-type mucus: it may become thinner and/or more liquid, creamy beadlike, et cetera, so you can chart an **M**, and the opening of the vagina will feel wet and slightly sticky, or most likely, it will just feel wet, so you can chart an **S** or **W**, respectively (here it is days 10, 11). Some women also note an odor that is characteristic of fertile mucus.

4. *S-type Mucus* Wet mucus that can be *stretched about 2.5 centimeters/1 inch*, causing a very wet sensation in the vagina, indicates fertile mucus. This mucus is charted (on line 3) by putting a **circle around an M** (here it is days 12, 13). You can indicate the wet vaginal sensation with a **W**.

5. *Peak Day* The Peak day (here it is day 13) is the last day that there is the slippery, wet, *stretchy* S-type mucus. The Peak day must be noted by **marking an X on the last circled M** (on line 3). It is not necessarily the day that you observe the greatest amount of mucus. *Charting this day correctly is essential to timing intercourse.*

6. *Change in Mucus Pattern* After the Peak day, the mucus

will either disappear or return to earlier characteristics (*not* S-type mucus). This change signifies that the previous day was the Peak day. You will have to record this for several cycles before you can begin to see a pattern and predict your Peak day.

The mucus change warns of the end of the fertile phase and the beginning of the post-ovulatory infertile phase, which begins after the fourth consecutive day of sticky, pasty mucus and/or dry sensations *after* the Peak day. You can indicate this on your chart by recording the numbers **1, 2, 3, 4** on the appropriate days (here you would record this on days 14 to 17).

Peak Day and Ovulation

Ovulation can occur anytime from three days before *the Peak day to three days* after the *Peak day*. Continue to chart your pattern even though you feel you have identified the Peak day. If wet mucus reappears, you may have identified the Peak day incorrectly or ovulation was delayed. Once your period starts, you have begun your next cycle and a new chart is used.

Charting Changes in the Cervix

You would use lines 5, 6 and 7 shown on the sample chart on page 113 to mark changes in the position and texture of your cervix. You should check your cervix at the same time each day, and, more specifically, at the same time each evening, so as not to disturb your mucus symptoms during the day.

First, wash your hands thoroughly for 15 seconds, using soap and warm water, to prevent any vaginal infection. **Do not use a lubricating substance**. If entering the vagina is difficult, use tap water to first wet your fingers. It is best to examine the cervix when both the bladder and rectum are empty. Pressure from either can alter the position of the cervix. Position yourself the same way each time you check. Standing is often easier.

Insert one or two fingers into the vagina, using gentle pressure to reach the cervix. You are using the same angle as you do when inserting a tampon. You will feel the firmer ridges of the vagina and then the smoother, rounder shape of the cervix. You may find it easier if you squat or stand with one foot on a stool. Ask yourself

1. Is it closed (●), like a little dimple, or open (○), like a small hole?
2. Is it easy to reach (low) or difficult to reach (high)?

On line 5, to show the position of the cervix as lower, you would chart a circle near the bottom of the space. As the cervix rises, you would mark the circle higher up the space, using the top of the area to show that the cervix is very high. Notice and chart if the cervix is open by using an "open" circle (○), or closed by making the circle solid (●). This is called the os diameter. Asking yourself

1. Is it firm (F), like the tip of a nose, or soft (S), like lips or the lobe of an ear?
2. Is it tilted (/) (your finger is hooked to reach it), or straight (|), (your finger reaches it easily)?

C e r v i x																															
Open/closed					●	●	●	●	○	○	○	○	○	○	●	●	●	●													5
Firm/soft					F	F	F	S	S	S	S	S	S	S	S	F	F	F	F												6
Tilt					/	/	/	/	/	/	I	I	I	I	I	/	/	/	/												7

You would chart these observations on lines 6 and 7 respectively, using the appropriate symbols. All of the underlined, second characteristics are signs of fertility or impending ovulation.

Charting Basal Body Temperature (BBT)

On the same fertility chart as you have been noting your cervical mucus and characteristics of the cervix, you would record your temperature readings every morning.

In order to take your basal body temperature (BBT), you must first purchase a BBT thermometer, which will cost about $10 to $15 at a drugstore. A normal thermometer used to determine fevers does not work because its graduations are not fine enough. The one I used was in Celsius degrees, but there are also Fahrenheit thermometer if you prefer. The charts provided in this book are in Celsius. **If you are using Fahrenheit, your charts should start at 96.9 °F and go up to 99.1 °F, in 1/10° increments.**

Take Your BBT Before You Get Out of Bed

Shake down the BBT thermometer and take your temperature as soon as you wake up, *before* you get up or move around. You must take it by the *same route* each time, whether it be orally for six to eight minutes, vaginally or rectally, for five minutes. (Note that the vaginal and rectal temperatures are usually 1 °C higher than the oral temperature.) Usually the temperature is between 36.2° and 36.4 °C/97.2° and 97.5 °F. Using a digital thermometer will make reading the results easier. Your temperature may be slightly higher during your period.

Please note that you must take your BBT at the same time every day and that you must have had one hour's rest before taking your temperature. The BBT must be taken when the body is at its most relaxed state. Your partner can be helpful in this regard to ensure the most accurate reading. For instance, let your partner answer your other children if they call for you right before you have to take your temperature.

Make sure you do not fall asleep or you may break the thermometer. If you work shifts, try to take your BBT after your normal bedtime. Being up for short periods each night will probably not have an adverse effect on your readings.

Record Your BBT (line 8)
Each day, put a dot on the chart corresponding to that correct day and degree (the BBT chart *begins* with line 8). If the mercury in the thermometer is between two lines, the lower one is charted. Shake down the thermometer. Draw a line connecting the dots .

Draw a Coverline
Sometimes the temperature can be higher during the menstrual period but it will drop down. Count the first six to ten days of low temperatures and draw a **coverline** just above the highest recorded temperature. A coverline is a horizontal line drawn just above the highest of the first six records of the BBT (e.g., if the highest temperature is 36.6 °C, draw the coverline between 36.6 °C and 36.7 °C) Line 9 shows an example of a coverline where the highest of the first six temperatures was 36.6 °C.

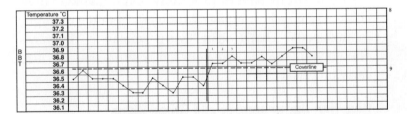

Determine Ovulation
A shift above the coverline indicates ovulation. Ovulation usually occurs when there is a drop in temperature and then a sharp increase followed by a temperature that remains around this same elevated level until the end of

the cycle. A true temperature shift occurs when three consecutive daily temperatures are at least 0.2 °C/0.2 °F above the previous six consecutive daily temperatures. Wait for three temperatures in a row to be recorded above the coverline to signify the beginning of the infertile phase. Draw a **vertical line** between the last low temperature and the sharp rise, and then record **1, 2, 3** to show the end of the fertile phase.

If the temperature rises above the coverline and then drops below, it may be a sign that ovulation has not occurred. This is called a **false high rise**. Wait until it goes above again before counting the three days. Sometimes a false high occurs when counting the ten days. It is not used to determine the coverline. The chart below is an example of a false high rise.

False High Rise

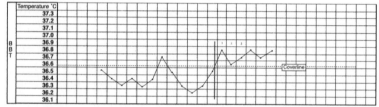

With lines joining the dots, you will be able to more clearly see your pattern of fertility and ovulation. Your chart may appear completely different from the example in this book. That's okay. Every woman is different. Should you forget to take your temperature one day, just carry on.

Charting Disturbances and Other Signs

As mentioned at the beginning of this chapter, there are many factors that may influence the signs of fertility. It is important to record any variables or disturbances you notice each day. These changes can alter your pattern and, subsequently, affect the way you read your chart.

Disturbances (lines 10, 11)

1. Intercourse Mark an X on the days that you have intercourse (see line 10 below). You must always record when you have intercourse because, as noted before, intercourse can change the appearance of cervical mucus.

Intercourse		X			X	X											X	X								10
Disturbances																										11
	FEVER																									

2. Other Disturbances Record all medications that are not usually taken (see line 11 above). (For example, I take a thyroid hormone every day and, therefore, would not note it on my charts.) Medications can alter the consistencey of your CM. Remember, temperatures go up and down for many reasons: alcohol, a late night, being up with a child, or the use of medication to reduce a fever. As I mentioned before, don't worry if you have these up-and-down recordings, which can happen before ovulation. Once you see the rise, you'll be able to pinpoint the drop.

Other disturbances include *illness, fever, stress, an ovarian cyst, diet changes, travel, oversleeping or fatigue, exercise, or alcohol,* et cetera.

Other Signs (line 12)

Finally, under the heading "Other Signs" (line 11 below), make note of any of the secondary signs of fertility, such as *abdominal pain, spotting, breast tenderness* or anything else you feel is relevant. Make up any abbreviations to suit you and add them to the legend. For example, I have coded abdominal pain as **AP**.

Other signs										AP															12

Supplementary Step: The Ovulation Kit

If you need further help to determine your time of fertility, you can purchase an ovulation kit at the drugstore. I have never used one and I find them to be expensive. However, many people have let me know that they were very helpful, in conjunction with charting, to determine when they ovulated.

The kit registers the luteinizing hormone (LH) surge that takes place before ovulation. Read carefully the instructions that come with your kit, as they will help you determine when to begin testing. You should attempt to start testing five to six days before you expect to ovulate. Test two times daily. Checking only once a day may mean you'll miss the LH surge. When testing in the evening, voiding should not have occurred within four hours of obtaining the sample. Reducing your liquid intake in the last two hours immediately before the procedure can help.

Again, I don't recommend using this as the sole method of determining ovulation, but it may be helpful in conjunction with my charting method.

To Prevent Unwanted Pregnancy

If you are relying solely on natural family planning as your form of birth control, it is important to know when you are fertile in order to prevent a pregnancy happening at the wrong time. There are two rules that will help: the alternate day rule and the twenty-one day rule.

Alternate-day Rule

When you are in the Basic Infertile Pattern (BIP), have intercourse on an every-other-day pattern; in other words, have intercourse one day, then skip a day before making love again. The reason for this rule is that, as mentioned, the presence of semen can confuse the CM readings.

Twenty-one-day Rule

The pre-ovulatory infertile phase begins on the first day of menstruation. Its length is found by subtracting 21 from the shortest of your six most recent and consecutive cycles. The cycles must be within the range of 25 to 37 days long, with no use of birth control pills. It is between 95 and 99 percent effective in avoiding pregnancy. For example, if the lengths of your last six cycles were 27, 29, 30, 26, 31, 34 days, subtract 21 from 26, since 26 is the shortest cycle: **26 - 21 = 5**. The first five days of the cycle (i.e. the first five days of menstruation) are considered infertile days.

Please remember that it *is* possible to become pregnant while on your period. Do not assume anything! If you have a very short pre-ovulatory phase—let's say four days—the colored discharge of your period may mask the fertile mucus signal. Thus, it is important to abstain from intercourse while any colored discharge is noted.

If any mucus is detected within the pre-ovulatory phase, you must consider yourself fertile.

Chapter 8
Interpreting Your Chart

Some charts are more difficult to read than others are. Recording your BBT for several months, comparing it with your observations of the cervix and the cervical mucus and using hindsight will make it easier to discern when ovulation happens.

What follows is an example of how to read and interpret your chart, and a discussion of some common problematic charts and their causes.

Martha's Fertility Chart

Let's look at Martha's Fertility Chart to pull everything together.

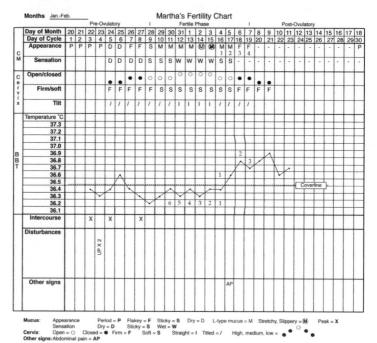

Martha's period began on January 20, which was day 1 of her cycle. She filled in the dates and charted a **P**. She menstruated for four days and then her CM felt dry for two days. Beginning on day three, Martha took her temperature orally for eight minutes prior to getting up and charted it. Note that on day 6 it went higher and then went down again. Under "Disturbances" she wrote **UP x2** because she had been up with one of her children during the night. After she counted six to ten low days (not counting day 6), she drew her coverline.

During the day, Martha checked her underpants and the toilet tissue. On days 7 and 8 she could scratch and flake off the discharge left on her underpants. But on day 9, it was sticky. Her cervix, although still closed, firm, and tilted, was harder to reach. The next day the cervix was higher still, softer and more open. Martha charted an **M** on that day, 10, because she found a creamy glob of discharge. She felt sticky at the opening of the vagina. On days 14 and 15, she could stretch the mucus 2.5 centimeters between her fingers. It was on day 16 that Martha no longer felt wet or slippery, and that she could not stretch the mucus. She put her **X** on the day before and then wrote a **1, 2, 3, 4** to mark the end of her fertile period.

Notice that her temperature stayed low until day 17 when it crossed the coverline and stayed there for three consecutive days. Martha found the temperature shift happened on day 17. There, too, she printed a **1** followed by a **2, 3** on days 18 and 19. Because ovulation usually occurs on the day before the shift, it would mean she ovulated on day 16. This appears to be the day after her Peak day. Fifteen days after her Peak day, her next period started.

Because Martha had charted her cycle for a year and a half, she was quite experienced at reading her signs. Thus, she did not keep charting after her post-ovulatory phase began. However, it is important to chart your cycles every day until your next period begins, until you are confident in recognizing each phase.

Causes for Discrepancies in Chart Interpretation

A woman using this natural method of reading her cycle will become very aware of disturbances or changes in her natural rhythm. There are many reasons for these irregularities.

Faulty Technique and Charting

The most common problem is faulty technique. There is no point recording temperature if it is not done properly. Use the same method each day, and take the same length of time for the temperature to register. Try to minimize disturbances that will affect the temperature and note disturbances as they occur.

Another problem is faulty charting. Make sure your records are consistent, truthful and accurately recorded.

Irregular Patterns

Somewhere along the line you may have a chart with an irregular pattern, often in the temperature section, even if no error was made in technique or charting. Often the chart will indicate a lack of ovulation, which can be traced to several factors. Below are a few of the more common irregularities in charts and corresponding sample charts.

1. Monophasic or Anovulatory Cycle Should the temperature remain on one level, it will indicate that there has been no ovulation. This is called a **monophasic** or **anovulatory cycle** (meaning a one-phase cycle). Bleeding is often lighter than usual and it is not a true period.

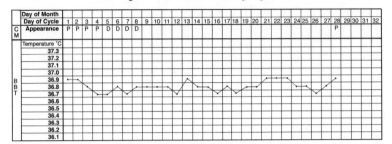

Monophasic or Anovulatory Cylce

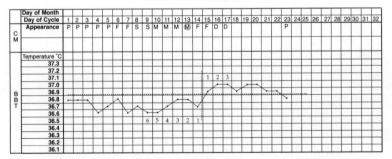

2. Short Luteal Phase A temperature that goes up and down in the post-ovulatory phase may indicate a problem with the woman's progesterone level. This is called a **short luteal phase**. Rather than being 12 to 16 days, the post-ovulatory phase lasts eight to ten days. When interpreting the chart and counting back 12 to 16 days from the start of her next period, the woman will notice that the temperature shift is in the "wrong" place. This is why the observation of the cervical mucus is so important and is the best indication of fertility. A short luteal phase may mean that fertilization is possible but implantation cannot occur.

Short Luteal Phase

3. Breast-feeding While a woman breast-feeds, she does not normally ovulate, and thus is 98 percent protected from pregnancy provided she is fully breast-feeding (i.e., no formula is being used at all, and menstruation has not returned). She can watch for her signs of fertility returning as she starts to introduce foods to her child and thus decrease the amount she breast-feeds.

While she is breast-feeding she will have a long phase of the BIP pattern of dryness. (Note that she is charting by the week, e.g, week 34, 35, 36, et cetera.) Temperature will swing and the cervix will remain low, firm, closed and tilted. Once she begins to decrease the number of breast-feeds she will start to notice a change in her mucus pattern from the BIP to periods of sticky or cloudy mucus and then back again. Her temperature may swing up and down while she is feeding a lot, but as she decreases the feeds she may be able to draw a coverline. The mucus is observed more and more frequently until she will see the slippery, clear, stretchy mucus leading to ovulation. As before, she will note the temperature shift. The post-ovulatory phase will begin after the fourth high temperature after the Peak day has been recorded. This phase may be a bit shorter than normal.

Breast-feeding

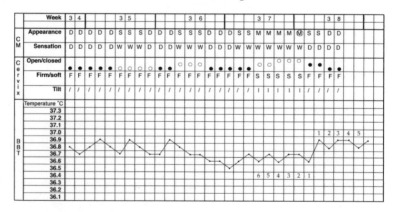

4. Premenstrual Syndrome (PMS) Prior to their periods, many women experience normal changes prior to their periods such as breast tenderness and irritability or mood swings. If the symptoms last a long time or are severe they may cause disruption in the woman's life physically, mentally and socially.

5. *Post Birth Control Pill* After going off the Pill, each woman's body may behave differently from another woman's, and differently each time she stops. It is advisable to wait and chart for three months to establish and understand the cyclic changes before getting pregnant. Irregularities commonly seen are

- Variations in cycle length and phases (e.g., short post-ovulatory phase of about eight to ten days; variations in the day that the key temperature shift occurs; cycles without ovulation).
- Erratic mucus pattern
- Effects on temperature (e.g., false high temperatures or the temperature and mucus signs do not correlate).

6. *Pre-menopausal Symptoms* As a woman approaches menopause, her fertility declines and ovulation can become irregular, resulting in irregular periods. The cervical mucus becomes reduced in quantity and loses its fertile quality in some cycles. Continuous dryness is usually noted. However, some women notice a constant, unchanging pattern of moistness, also a BIP. With the woman's BBT, she may notice variations in the temperature shift depending on the length of her cycles (which may vary a lot), and some cycles where there is no shift (monophasic/anovulatory).

Bleeding may go from scant to heavy. A true period will be recognized because it follows ovulation, which is preceded by a temperature shift 12 to 14 days earlier. Periods will become shorter, lighter and farther apart. This is normal. Should they become closer together, longer and heavier, a woman should consult her physician. The same is true if she has vaginal bleeding more than one year after her last period.

Practice Interpreting a Fertility Chart

The following fertility chart is one on which you can practice, using the following steps to interpret the chart. The answers are found in Appendix B.

Practice Chart

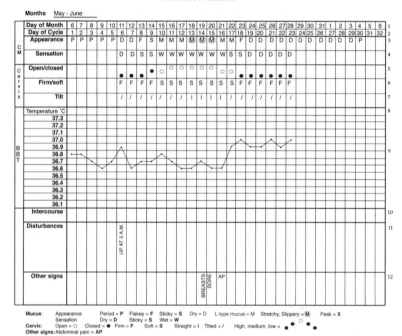

1. Determine the length of the cycle.

2. BBT Chart

a) Determine the day of the temperature shift. Count the first six low temperatures and draw a coverline above the highest dot of the six. Count three high temperatures. Draw a verticle line between the last low temperature and the first high temperature and extend the line up past the top line, "Day of Month".

b) Check for factors (stress, illness, medications, sleep problems) that may influence the temperature.

c) Identify the first day of the post-ovulatory infertile phase.

3. Mucus Pattern

a) Determine the length of the period.

b) Identify the first appearance of mucus.

c) Identify the pre-ovulatory infertile phase. Look for the Basic Infertile Pattern (BIP) of non-changing mucus, or dry, flaky mucus and/or dry vaginal sensations.

d) Identify the fertile phase, days of wet mucus, especially stretchy mucus. Mark the Peak day with an **X**. Number **1,2,3,4** on the four days after the Peak day.

e) Identify the post-ovulatory infertile phase.

f) Correspond the temperature chart with the mucus chart to identify the probable day of ovulation.

4. Changes in Cervix
a) Identify the infertile phase (low, firm, closed, tilted).
b) Identify the fertile phase (high, soft, open, straight).

5. Other Indicators: identify other signs such as abdominal pain, et cetera, to determine ovulation.

Chapter 9
Putting the Theory to Work:
Timing Intercourse

The average of North American births recorded each year over the past 20 years shows that 51 percent of baby's born were male and 49 percent were female. Chances are almost even for a girl to be conceived as are the chances for a boy to be conceived. This chapter will teach you how to significantly increase those chances either way, primarily by timing sexual intercourse.

Let's review the genetics of conception. Each sperm cell contains either an X or Y chromosome. The X chromosome will result in a girl baby. This female sperm has a large oval head lives longer and is much more hardy, or resistant, to stress, cold, chemicals and so on. The Y chromosome produces a boy. The male sperm has a rounder head, is smaller, more compact and swims much faster than the female sperm. However, the male sperm is not as strong as the female sperm. It likes a more alkaline environment while the female sperm can tolerate a more acidic one. Keep these characteristics in mind and you will understand more easily the basic principles in influencing the conception of a child of either sex.

One more reminder: As in all other stages of this process, it is strongly suggested that you use some form of birth control, either condoms or the natural family planning method, until you are ready to conceive a child. You and your partner may want to practice timing intercourse a few times before you attempt to conceive, just to ensure that all of the proper steps are in place.

Trying for a Boy: Intercourse at Ovulation

Of all the animals, the boy is the most unmanageable.

—Plato

When trying to conceive a boy, your primary goal is to create a situation where a sperm carrying the Y chromosome reaches and fertilizes the egg first. Logically, the faster male sperm will most likely be the first to reach and penetrate the egg if you have intercourse at or near the time of ovulation. At this time the secretions are more alkaline, more favorable for male sperm survival, and the egg will be moving closer to the uterus, which reduces the distance the sperm have to travel.

Sperm Count

A **high sperm count** is beneficial for conceiving a boy. If male sperm are not very hardy and die off more easily in the vagina, then having as many as possible will increase the chances of conceiving a boy. "But," you say, "that means there will be more female sperm, too!" Yes, you're right; but the male sperm, with their speed, will get there first!

Studies show that tight-fitting clothes, such as tight jeans or jockey shorts, increase the temperature of the scrotum, thereby killing the sperm cells, especially the males, and lowering the overall (male and female) sperm count. Hot tubs or hot work places can also have a similar effect. Stress can decrease the count, as can high altitudes, illness, toxic chemicals, smoking, radiation and recreational drugs.

To help boost the count, the man can keep the genitals cool by wearing loose-fitting clothes, such as boxer shorts and loose trousers. Men can also help by sponging their testicles with cool or cold water. Because spermatogenesis takes about 70 days, sponging for three months prior to attempting to conceive would be best. One "drug" that is helpful is caffeine. Because it helps to boost the count, it is beneficial for you, Dad, to drink a cup or two of coffee or tea 15 to 30 minutes before intercourse.

Condoms

It is essential to use a condom until you are ready to try for a boy. Better yet, abstain completely from sex until the woman ovulates. **Abstaining** from ejaculation for four days will allow the sperm count to be at its optimum. This is especially beneficial to men who have a low male sperm count or who have a low sperm count overall. Continue to use a condom after the trying, until the woman's fertile period has definitely passed.

Timing Intercourse for a Boy

With reference to the woman's chart, have intercourse between the time you believe to be the last low temperature, and the morning on which you note the sharp rise. The rise should coincide with the days the woman is experiencing Peak day signs but you will want to wait until *after* the Peak day before having intercourse. **The goal is to time intercourse as close to ovulation as possible.**

1. Use All Three Charting Methods When my husband and I were planning our third child, I was observing only my cervical mucus. My cycle always began 16 days after my Peak day, so I felt that I probably ovulated perhaps two days later than the Peak day. Two of my friends estimated their time of ovulation in a similar way. All three couples timed their lovemaking for the third day after marking an X. We all had boys. I was not using the BBT method—with our two young daughters, I never got any sleep! Perhaps if I had charted my temperature, I would have seen the time of ovulation more clearly. Therefore, I recommend using all three methods for greater accuracy.

2. If Using an Ovulation Kit If you are using an ovulation kit, test twice a day between 11:00 a.m. and 3:00 p.m., and between 5:00 p.m. and 10:00 p.m. Space at least ten hours between tests (noon and 10:00 p.m. are best). Wait 12 hours after first detecting your LH surge before having intercourse. This reference will be understood more clearly once you have read your kit instructions. Make sure you wait for the slippery mucus!

Position
A deeper penetration, putting the sperm nearer the cervix by "spooning", or entering the vagina from behind, is best.

Alkalinity
An alkaline envirmonent in the vagina is a more favorable condition for the male sperm. One way to increase the alkalinity is for the woman to time her orgasm just before or at the same time as her partner's. This is not critical, but it may be helpful. Another method that is no longer recommended is the use of a basic baking-soda douche. This method is not advised unless recommended by a doctor, because the use of douches has been linked to ectopic pregnancies and pelvic inflammatory disease (PID).

Trying for a Girl: Intercourse Before Ovulation

The female of the species is more deadly than the male.
— Rudyard Kipling

When trying for a girl, you want to have more female than male sperm cells awaiting the arrival of the egg. The larger, hardier, but slower female sperm will be more apt to fertilize the egg if intercourse occurs *more than a day in advance* of ovulation. At this time, the secretions in the vagina are more acidic and harmful to the male sperm, and the journey to the egg is long. By the time the egg is released, the male sperm have either died en route from the harsher conditions, or perished while waiting for the egg to burst out of the ovary. Meanwhile, the slow-swimming female sperm can survive for a longer period and arrive in time to fertilize the egg.

Sperm Count

A **low sperm count** has been associated with the conception of females. Clothing that causes the temperature of the scrotum to be greater than 36 °C/96.8 °F significantly lowers the count. The only way it is safe for a man to try to lower his sperm count is by wearing tighter underwear or a jock strap during the day **for only five days and no more** before attempting to conceive. And, as mentioned before, the more often a man ejaculates, the fewer sperm there are in his semen.

Condoms

In this case, the lack of! Don't use a condom when you are trying for a girl. Have intercourse, if possible, daily from when the bleeding stops until and including the cut-off day (five days before ovulation), but **only if the man has**

a high sperm count. After the cut-off day, abstain from sex until four days after ovulation.

Timing Intercourse for a Girl

Again, determining the time of ovulation is important and you will time intercourse to occur four, three or two days before ovulation. When observing your cervical mucus, do not have intercourse on the Peak day or for four days after.

1. The Importance of the BBT Graph   If you have a **regular cycle**, look at the day you normally record your last low temperature and subtract three. For example, if you have your last low on day 14, schedule the date of your last intercourse for day 11.

When your cycles are irregular, check your last four to six cycles and either take the earliest date of ovulation and subtract three days or take the number of days in the shortest cycle and subtract 14 to get the earliest probable ovulation date in any month. Subtract three days from that total. This final answer is the last day you should have intercourse until you are definitely in the post-ovulatory infertile phase (e.g., if the shortest cycle is 40 days, you subtract 14 to get 26. Then subtract 3 days to get day 23. This means that day 23 of your cycle is the last day you can safely have intercourse until the post-ovulatory phase.)

Your aim is to have intercourse as far before ovulation as possible and still conceive. Try five days prior. If you don't conceive, try four days, then three days in the subsequent cycles. If you still are not pregnant, **try two days before but no closer**.

2. *If Using an Ovulation Kit* If you are using an ovulation kit, stop having intercourse at least one day before the LH surge. Obviously, the day before your surge may be hard to figure out without the help of your charts. Again, I strongly recommend the use of all three methods in the chart, using the ovulation kit as a supplementary method.

Position
Shallow penetration, where the couple is face to face, with the man on top (missionary position), is most beneficial. Because the sperm must travel through the acidic secretions of the vagina there is a better chance that the male sperm will die and more female sperm will get through. If you have a tipped uterus, lie quietly on your stomach for 15 minutes after making love. Place a pillow under your upper thighs to elevate your legs a little—this helps the sperm get into the cervix.

Alkalinity
A less alkaline environment is favorable for female sperm. Ways to decrease the alkalinity including timing the woman's orgasm *after* the man's. Again, douches are not necessary except when prescribed by a doctor.

Summary
For a boy
- Have intercourse at or just after ovulation.
- Abstain from sex until ovulation to have a high sperm count.
- When the stretchy, slippery S-type mucus is evident, have intercourse once.
- Keep the man's genitals cool by wearing loose-

fitting underpants and trousers.

• Try for deeper penetration by "spooning", or entering the vagina from behind.

For a girl

• Have intercourse every day up to five days before ovulation, using no condoms.

• Do not have intercourse again until after the fertile period.

• Keep the man's genitals warm by wearing tighter-fitting underpants (no more than five days before intercourse).

• Try for more shallow penetration, making love with the man on top and both partners facing each other in the missionary position, so that the male sperm have farther to swim in a more hostile environment.

Part Four

Correspondence and Comments

I often remind my own children that when they are deciding whether or not to do something and there is a hesitation, an "iffy" feeling or guilt, then the decision becomes a "no" until the feelings become positive. The same is true for deciding to have another baby simply because you are hoping for a particular sex. If there is hesitation about wanting the "wrong" sex, then it is not the right choice.

Over the years, I have received many calls and letters from people interested in the topic of sex preselection and looking to make the right choice for themselves. Sometimes they had questions about the method or where they could find more information. Often, the couple had already decided to try to choose the sex of their baby, but they needed to learn how to read their cycles. At other times, I would hear about a new baby who had been born and the parent's appreciation of my assistance. I thought some of their stories would make interesting reading and that some of the questions may be similar to ones you have.

Chapter 10
Some of the Stories

Over the past few years, I have contacted many people who have used my technique. I asked them three questions. Did they use the method to predetermine the sex of a child? Were they successful? Could they tell me about their experience? Of the few who weren't successful, they said that they had not followed my technique properly, but when they looked back at their charts they saw that the sex of their baby confirmed the method.

In 1996 one woman wrote to me about her frustrations with other methods:

As the mother of four daughters, aged six and under, I can only dream of having a son. I love my girls very much and feel guilty for not being satisfied but I can't talk myself out of it. I've already tried everything: prayer, temperature method, baking-soda douches, timing, et cetera. But I feel it is worth trying again. I just thought I'd tell you that my cycle happens every 29 to 32 days and that mid-cycle cramps can occur up to a week prior to ovulation so any extra tips besides your book would be welcome. —H.C.

And then after my advice, in 1997, she wrote back:

Just a quick note to let you know the outcome of my last pregnancy. It's a boy! It's really nice to have a son after four daughters and I'll know I won't have to wonder "if" for the rest of my life. I truly feel I have the perfect family now and am very happy. Although I didn't follow all your suggestions, I particularly paid attention to the part of waiting two to three days after you think for sure it is the Peak day.... Coincidence or not, I still give the glory to the Lord above for another healthy baby. And after years of praying, I have to think of the adage, God helps those who help themselves. I want to thank you for your part in it. —H.C.

Many people who are planning their first child do not consider sex selection. Most often, the couple has had at least one child before looking for information on preselection. However, this next letter demonstrates that even first-time parents will consider it if the information is available.

Just a short note of appreciation for your information on choosing the sex of your baby. We gave much thought to what sex we would try for, it being out first child. We decided on a boy. The very first month, three days after I had charted an X on my chart, our son was conceived. We had told our friends and family that we had followed your advice and tried for a boy. At first they laughed but now they seem quite convinced. Thanks again. —L.C.

The letters and calls I have received about successes have been overwhelming. The couples who have written to me come from various cultural backgrounds, personal belief systems, and with particular reasons for choosing their baby's sex. These are just a sample.

My husband and I used your advice to try for both our son and our daughter. Although we knew we would be happy with whatever we were blessed with, we had wanted a child of each sex because we thought it would be "neat" and we only wanted two children. We wanted to find some way to increase our chances that was a natural way. We do not agree with all this information and talk about genetic engineering. Your method is natural and it worked! —D.K.

We used your advice to have the order we were hoping for. We wanted a boy to be the oldest in the family. Then we wanted a girl. Finally, because my husband has two sisters and I have one sister, we wanted another boy. We were successful for all three! Thank you so much. —W.A.

We had a young daughter and were hoping to have a son. I am from Nepal. In my parents' generation, it was important to have a boy. I think it is not so much in my generation. But we wanted one of each. My daughter is seven and a half and my son is now 18 months! You were right! —M.J.

We were successful in having a boy 11 months after the first normal period I had following breast-feeding. We already had a son and wanted another child of the same sex, very close in age if possible. I breast-fed for five months, charted my cycles and now have boys who are 18 months apart. —G.C.

We were so excited that it worked! My husband is one of nine children. He has four brothers and four sisters. None of his brothers has a son. Only three of his four sisters have children, and each has a boy. We have fifteen nieces and three nephews and now our son has joined the family! Thank you! —R.L.

My husband and I had two boys and wanted a girl. It was really easy and simple. We thought about how we conceived the first two, when I was ovulating and using the "from behind" position. Then we did it differently—before I ovulated and using a different position like you said. It worked and we had our daughter. —S.J.

Our daughter was born. She was just so wonderful! We always wanted to have two children and we wanted another girl. We hoped with two girls that they would grow to be really good friends, and it would be easier economically if they were the same sex—you know, hand-me-downs and shared interests. We conceived our first daughter instantly. It took us about four months to get pregnant with our second child. But it worked! By the way, I shared your method with my cousin and it worked for her, too! —K.L.

Some people were successful but still skeptical:

Yes, we had our boy—but I think it was purely chance. —P.S.

Others had success even using just part of the method:

We had three girls and were trying for a boy. We only relied on plotting the temperature and didn't use any other suggestions. We had another girl. —V.E.

And a few couples who did not have success realized it was because they didn't apply my technique fully:

We did not get the sex we were hoping for but your method was correct! We were trying for a boy and using the ovulation kit. We had intercourse when I noticed the LH surge. I learned later that, when there is the LH surge, sometimes it can last two days before it fades out. If I had waited until it had faded, it would have been better I think. After seeing the LH surge, maybe wait 24 to 50 hours. Also, use a combination of two or three methods, such as the kit and mucus charting, to better determine ovulation. —J.K.

"J" is quite correct in her musings. Ovulation kits register the surge of the luteinizing hormone (LH) that takes place just before ovulation. Intercourse at this point should result in a girl. This is why my technique encourages using all three of the natural ways to determine ovulation.

And a few couples tried my technique without success. In 1995, one woman wrote to me:

I hope to have a boy. I presently have three beautiful daughters but for my next child I would like to have a boy. —D.T.

And in 2000 she wrote back:

We tried using your advice. I charted my cycle for a while. But we now have four beautiful daughters. Both my husband and I have brothers and sisters who have all had sons and daughters. Obviously our four girls were meant to be. They are wonderful. —D.T.

Another couple tried, but had difficulty using the method. Yet, like the others, they were still happy with their child. After all, a new baby, whatever the sex, is a miracle.

My husband and I had a son and were hoping to have a girl so that we could have the experience of raising both. I was pretty sure when ovulation was happening, although I couldn't feel when the cervix was open. I used the temperature method and tried to go by mucus, too, trying to have a girl. We tried four days before I thought I'd ovulate and didn't get pregnant, then three days, then two days and I was pregnant. But I had a boy.

My husband is one of two boys also. We love both our sons dearly and they are such good playmates. Maybe that's why we had a boy! —M.N.

Unfortunately, not everyone agrees with the concept of gender preselection. At the Parents Show in Toronto a few years ago, a woman, angry that I would "dare promote such a thing", reproached me. Another time, a doctor and the editor of an obstetrician/gynecologist magazine, said that natural sex selection was wrong because it was rather like playing God. This comment amazed me— especially from a doctor! When I think of the knowledge this book imparts about the workings of our bodies and what we can do when we understand some basic physiology— things as simple as preventing or planning a pregnancy— and compare it to the wonderful technology that we have today that enables a two-pound, premature baby to survive or a life to be saved through micro-surgery, I would question which one could be most likened to playing God. I believe that we have been created with minds for us to use fully, and that doing so has given us opportunities and choices that we never had before. I am as thankful for the miraculous technologies which enhance and prolong life as I am for the basic knowledge I have learned about the miracle of reproduction.

This following letter, however, has a different viewpoint.

The fact that you are an RN with experience in public health and prenatal teaching doesn't mean you have a social conscience or respect for Mother Nature. I am not assuming that you are cold-hearted and misguided—but anyone who plays "God" with Mother Nature has been misguided somewhere.

Choosing to choose your baby's sex shows that you cannot accept life's miracles that we are blessed with and really don't deserve a child. You should put your energy into something worthwhile. Don't fool with Mother Nature! —G.J.

In the seven years that I have publicly endorsed this method, there were only three people who disagreed with the concept and let me know. I do respect their right to an opinion, even if it differs with mine. Fortunately though, this is the rare exception rather that the rule.

Finally, I'd like to end with one of the most positive letters I've received so far. This lovely note from a father touches on so many of the thoughts and feelings many have had as parents.

Wonderful dreams of snuggling and loving a little bundle of joy had long been part of my wife's routine, so you can just imagine her excitement as we discussed plans to begin our family. Just a little scared, we shared our common views and thoughts on health issues, parenting and hoped, above all, that the miracle of childbirth would bless us with a healthy baby.

At the time, my dreams (which were proven quite silly after the birth of my second child, a daughter) were not about snuggling a baby or holding a bundle of joy. I dreamed about mountain biking, rock climbing and playing sports with our child and, for some reason, that child was a boy. Perhaps I was just afraid that all the walls in our house would be pink! You can imagine my excitement when I learned through a friend that your advice could help us understand the process of conception process better and perhaps naturally allow us to help Mother Nature out a little.

Once my wife and I were comfortable with our new understanding of the factors that contributed to determining gender, we set out to try and have not only a beautiful, healthy baby to snuggle and love, but also a boy to some day round out my adventure racing team (in my dreams of course). On October 5, 1993, we were blessed with a beautiful little boy.

Several years later, as my wife proudly displayed the new clothes (all great deals!) she had purchased for our son, it became clear to me that she wanted some day to be dressing a little girl in new baby clothes. It was my wife's turn, and we laid plans to complete our family.

We were challenged with many medical troubles through-out my wife's difficult pregnancy, but through some miracle and a little help from you, we were overjoyed to introduce our son to his new baby sister on April 16, 1997.

Our experience as parents has altered some of the views and opinions we shared seven years ago. My wife realizes that our daughter, even at three years old, would rather choose her own clothes to wear, and I realize that even if I did have an adventure competition team, it would be stronger with both my son and my daughter as members. You truly touched our lives and helped us enter the parenting world with the family of our dreams. Thank you. —J. C.

Chapter 11
Questions and Answers

Q. I am presently on the Pill. How long should I wait after going off it before trying to choose the sex of my next baby?
A. Wait at least three months so that your body will have had a chance to return to its normal cycle. This time will give you a chance to practice determining when you ovulate.

Q. Will getting pregnant one month after going off the Pill cause abnormalities in the fetus?
A. No. Many women revert right back to their normal cycles after they go off the Pill. The Pill is made of artificial versions of a woman's natural hormones and it doesn't contain anything that can harm the developing embryo.

Q. Must we use a condom or may we use the withdrawal method when not wanting to become pregnant?
A. The answer is a definite no. Withdrawal, or coitus interruptus, is not a method of birth control. The slippery fluid on the end of the penis contains sperm. Even having just the tip of the penis touch the outside of the vagina can result in a pregnancy. Also, even though the male doesn't ejaculate, some semen comes out of the penis through sexual excitement. Recently, I read a good saying: "There is a word for people who depend on that particular method (withdrawal) of birth control—parents."

Q. Will using lubricated condoms have any effect on my readings?

A. The only lubrication I advise is water. Any other kind, including water-based lubrication used with latex condoms or K-Y Jelly, may confuse your CM data.

Q. Can I use the rhythm method to determine when I am fertile?

A. The rhythm method only works if the woman has a regular, 28-day cycle, and very few women do. In this method, the woman counts 12 to 14 days from the start of her period to determine when she is most fertile, which, according to the rhythm method will always be day 14 of her cycle. The method is often unreliable because it is not the pre-ovulatory phase but only the post-ovulatory phase that is consistent. This means that she can only count back 12 to 14 days from the start of her next period to determine the fertile period.

Furthermore, the rhythm method works only if she has a 28-day cycle: **28 - 14 = 14**. However, if she were to have a 36 day cycle, **36 - 14 = 22**, she will misjudge and be fertile eight days later than she planned. The same is true for a shorter cycle such as one with 21 days, **21 - 14 = 7**. Oops, missed again! Research shows over and over that the most effective and reliable indication of fertility for women with is the apperance of the clear, stretchy S-type cervical mucus. Not only is the rhythm method often inaccurate but it doesn't take into account the fertile mucus.

Q. Do I really need to keep a chart?

A. Yes, you really do. Comparing the fertility signs of each cycle will make you more certain of when you ovulate, a certainty that is vital for knowing when to have intercourse. Don't trust your memory to record all the data that helps you pinpoint ovulation!

Q. Doesn't charting all the fertility signs and following all of the method's rules take the spontaneity out of lovemaking?
A. Yes and no. You do have to obey the rules and be diligent in keeping your chart. However, in each cycle the infertile phase is a period when you can't get pregnant— you're lovemaking can be as spontaneous as you wish!

Q. How long do you recommend that I keep my charts before "going for it"? Is there any rule of thumb?
A. Chart for at least three cycles, and then keep charting until you are confident in reading them and pinpointing ovulation. The only rule of thumb is to wait until you're ready to "go for it".

Q. If I understand my signs, will I be able to know if I have an infection?
A. Definitely! Understanding the normal rhythms of your body will help you to recognize any unusual or troublesome signs.

Q. Are there any drugs that help choose the sex of a baby? If so, do you recommend them?
A. I don't know of any drugs that help determine the sex of a baby. I would be wary of any drug that purports to help with sex selection. In any event, you should follow your doctor's advice with any drug that you are using, and once you conceive, you shouldn't take any drugs unless prescribed by a physician.

Q. How long does the egg live if it is not fertilized?
A. The egg will normally live 12 to 24 hours.

Q. How many days in each cycle are most couples fertile?

A. A male is fertile as long as he is producing sperm and semen of the correct consistency and quantity, the reproductive ducts and channels are clear for the passage of the reproductive fluids, and the penis can become erect and ejaculation is possible. A woman is fertile a few days before her Peak day and a few days after, when the fertile mucus is present and within one or two days of ovulation (the egg lives for 12 to 24 hours after ovulation). A recent report states that sperm may live for up to six days in the woman's body, as long as they are swimming in fertile mucus. Therefore, a couple may be fertile between three and six days each cycle.

Q. Is it possible to conceive without producing the fertile mucus?

A. Research shows that fertile mucus must be present in order for conception to occur. The mucus is necessary to nurture the sperm and to assist the movement of the sperm.

Q. Sometimes I can feel dry all day, but when my partner and I start to make love, I feel wet. Is this fertile mucus?

A. Your fertile mucus may have started. However, it could also be the mucus that is secreted upon sexual excitement to lubricate the vagina and make intercourse easier. You should always be aware of your mucus, and have checked your mucus several times before you have even thought of making love. Once you have charted for a few months and looked at your pattern, you will recognize the difference between the lubricating mucus of excitement and fertile mucus.

Q. I feel as if I am interested more in making love when the mucus is the fertile type. Is this true or am I just imagining it?
A. No, you are not imagining it. We have been created beautifully so that we will keep our species going. The mucus, being so slippery, makes intercourse easier and it gives you the same lubricated feeling as when you are sexually aroused. You may even detect that the fertile mucus has a different odor. Your body is signaling that it is fertile and ready for procreation.

Q. Sometimes there is a bit of blood in my panties a couple of weeks after my period. Am I having a little period?
A. No. The red-tinged mucus you may find between periods is called spotting and can occur close to ovulation. It is most likely caused by a surge of hormones at the time of ovulation, bringing up the estrogen level enough to cause some light bleeding. While there is a little blood loss, spotting is not a period.

Q. Why does the temperature rise at ovulation?
A. The secretion of progesterone, a hormone released at ovulation, causes the increase in temperature.

Q. How would you know if you had a tipped uterus?
A. You would not be able to feel it. A doctor would have to determine the position of your uterus by doing an internal examination.

Q. I have a tipped uterus. Should I try a different method?
A. No. The method is the same. However, it may help to lie quietly on your stomach, and place a pillow under your upper thighs to elevate your hips a bit. Remain in this position for for 15 minutes after intercourse, to help the sperm cells enter the cervix.

Q. Does having twins contradict the method for having a girl or a boy?

A. For identical twins, one fertilized egg splits apart resulting in two babies of the same sex. The theory behind timing intercourse for a girl or a boy holds because it is one egg that is initally fertilized. For fraternal twins, two eggs are released around the same time. The fertilization of both of these eggs will result in two babies of either the same or different sexes. The sex-selection theory still holds when the twins are the same sex. However, twins of different sexes presents more of a puzzle. Perhaps intercourse occurred after the release of one egg and before the release of the second.

Q. Can I use the method when I am breast-feeding?

A. When you are breast-feeding, your hormones remain at a level similar to pregnancy. You are 98 percent protected from becoming pregnant because you generally do not ovulate when breast-feeding. Once you begin to introduce solid foods, you will produce less breast milk because the baby will not be demanding as much. At this time, your hormone levels will change: you may start to ovulate, your periods may resume, and you may be able to become pregnant. Obviously, if you are not fertile, you cannot use the method to help you conceive a child of any sex. Because your readings will be irratic, you cannot use the method as a reliable form of birth control when you are fully breast-feeding. (I suggest the use of condoms or another method of birth control as a safeguard.)

However, if you want, you can continue charting while you are breast-feeding. You will have a long phase of infertility, noticing the Basic Infertile Pattern (BIP) of dryness or scant, sticky mucus. It may seem that sometimes the mucus is turning almost fertile and then returning to infertile. Your BBT will show a swinging pattern and your cervix will remain low, firm, closed and tilted. Once you are weaning your child, and begin to ovulate, you will be able to start charting and interpreting your signs as you did before pregnancy.

Q. *Are mannerisms inherited?*
A. Some scientists feel that mannerisms are learned behaviors: children will copy each other or their parents. Others suspect that mannerisms are passed on through genes. Scientists have observed that identical twins separated at birth will display similar mannerisms, which it is felt must come from their genetic makeup rather than environmental influences. The theory has yet to be proven.

Q. *If the embryo is "half dad", why does the mother's body not reject it, as with organ transplants?*
A. It is thought that the reason is simply that the 23 chromosomes from the mother must be enough for the mother's body to identify the embryo, which is why she does not reject it.

Q. *I have heard that we all start out as girls. Is that true?*
A. For six to seven weeks after conception, the sex of the fetus remains "in limbo". The embryo has undeveloped testes and ovaries. In male embryos, it seems that a chemical signal is sent from a gene on the Y chromosome to the testes. When the testes receive this signal they are stimulated to develop the penis and scrotum. Female development is then suppressed.

Q. *I know the sperm are really small. Can I see the egg?*
A. The egg is visible to the naked eye. It is very, very

small though, about 0.014 centimeters or 1/175 of an inch in diameter, and it weighs 1/20 of a millionth of an ounce. Sperm can only be seen under a microscope. Each one is 0.005 centimeter or 1/500 of an inch and weighs 1/90,000 the weight of the egg.

Q. Why does the man produce so many sperm when only one is needed?
A. Many sperm are needed for three reasons. First, the nature of the journey to the egg is a very hazardous one for sperm. Some die before they enter the vagina, while others fall out of the woman when she stands up. Approximately only 5 percent of the sperm will survive and make it to the cervix. The inside of the vagina is acidic and very hostile to sperm, which prefers an alkaline environment. Many die, despite the chemicals in the semen that try to neutralize some of the acidity. A second reason for the large numbers of sperm is that once inside the female reproductive tract, many of the sperm will go the wrong way and enter the fallopian tube to where no egg has been released. A third reason is that, although only one sperm enters the egg, the efforts of all the others are needed as their waving tails help to propel the egg along the tube.

Amazing, Don't You Think?

A study was done in Nigeria based upon the theory that a single act of intercourse at the Peak resulted in a boy, while intercourse around the time of the mucus change before the Peak, with abstinence until after the fertile phase produced a girl. Dr. Leonie McSweeney coordinated the study and reported that 310 couples achieved success in preselection of a boy. Four couples failed. Success in preselection of a girl occurred with 90 couples. Two couples failed. Amazing results? Not 100 percent by any means, but worthy of note!

There are no guarantees in life, and this book does not guarantee results. Your success will be determined to a large degree by your commitment to following the method diligently. That you are willing to and may play a part in determining the sex of your baby is exciting!

Congratulations on taking the first step in learning more about your and your partner's body and health. Perhaps you are deciding to start a family or taking steps to add to your family. Best of luck! You will be very fortunate, no matter what you have!

Bibliography

Bennett, Neil G., ed. *Sex Selection in Children*. New York: Academic Press, 1981.

Billings, Dr. Evelyn and Westmore, Anne. *The Billings Method Controlling Fertility Without Drugs or Devices*. New York: Random House, 1980.

Chesterman-Phillips, Hazel. *Choose the Sex of Your Baby —The Natural Way*. London: Bloomsbury Publishing, 1997.

Haney, Daniel Q. "What Makes a Boy or a Girl? Scientists May Have the Answer". *The Oregonian*. Assoc. Press, December 23, 1987.

Hilgers, Thomas W., et al. *The Ovulation Method of Natural Family Planning Book One*. Omaha, Nebraska: Creighton University Natural Family Planning and Research Center, 1982.

Kass-Annese, Barbara R.N., C.N.P. and Danzer, Hal M.D. *The Fertility Awarenss Workbook*. Atlanta, Georgia: Printed Matter, Inc., 1986.

Langendoen, Sally R.N. and Proctor, William. *The Preconception Gender Diet*. New York: M. Evans and Co. Ltd., 1982.

Martin, Lori. "Your Child's Sex—Can You Choose?". *Parents*. October 1981, p.72.

Bibliography

McCarthy, John J. Jr., M.D. and Martin, Mary Catherine M.S.N., Ph.D. *Fertility Awareness*. Alexandria, VA: The Human Life and Natural Family Planning Foundation, 1982.

Parenteane, Suzanne M.D. *Planning Your Family the S-T Way*. Ottawa: Serena Canada, 1987.

Shettles, Landrum B. M.D., Ph.D. and Rorvik, David M. "How to Choose the Sex of Your Baby". *Family Circle*. March 6, 1984, p.34.

Shettles, Landrum B. M.D., Ph.D. and Rorvik, David M. *How to Choose the Sex of Your Baby: The Method Best Supported by the Scientific Evidence* (newly revised). New York: Double Day, 1989.

Snowden, Robert and Elizabeth. *The Gift of A Child*. London: George Allen and Unwin (Publishers) Ltd., 1984.

Sullivan, Walters. "New Ways Devised to Pick Child's Sex". *New York Times*. September 23, 1987.

Tilton, Nan and Todd and Gaylen Moore. *In Vitro Fertilization*. New York: Doubleday, 1985

Verny, T. and Kelly, J. *The Secret Life of the Unborn Child*. New York: Summit Books, 1981.

Whelan, E. *Boy or Girl?* Indianapolis: Bobbs-Merrill Co., 1977.

Whelan, E. *Boy or Girl?* New York: Bobbs-Merrill Co., Inc., 1984

Young, Dr. J Martin. *How to Have a Boy A Step-by-Step Guide to Scientifically Maximize Your Chances of Conceiving a Son*. Amirillo, Texas: Young Ideas Publishing Division, 1995.

Young, Dr. J Martin. *How to Have a Girl A Step-by-Step Guide to Scientifically Maximize Your Chances of Conceiving a Daughter*. Amirillo, Texas: Young Ideas Publishing Division, 1995.

Internet Sources
"A Woman's Way to Health Trying to get Pregnant? Causes of Infertility in Women".
www.bayfront.org/explore/trying to/causesw.html, Health Adventure, 1997

"Artificial Insemination".
http://www.fertilitext.org/artinsem.htm

"Choose the Sex of Your Baby: Recent Study Says Sperm Cells Can Be Sorted".
http://wcco.com/news/stories/news-980909-075020.html, September 9, 1998.

"In Vitro Fertilization (IVF)".
http://www.fertilitext.org/ivf.htm

Garcia, Kathy. "The Astrology of Fertility".
http://atlantisrising.com/issue7/ar7topastrol.html

"Ancient Chinese Birth Gender Chart".
http://www.mypage.direct.ca/j/jfeng/gender.htm

Glossary

acidic — a sour or sharp chemical substance, the opposite of an alkaline

afterbirth — the expelled placenta

alkaline — having a salt base; the opposite of an acid

amniocentesis — the withdrawing of amniotic fluid from inside the uterus of a pregnant woman

amniotic fluid — the fluid found inside the amniotic sac that cushions the developing fetus

amniotic sac — the membranous sac surrounding the developing fetus, inside the uterus

anovulatory cycle — a menstrual cycle in which ovulation does not occur (also called monophasic)

anus — the opening to the rectum

artificial insemination — the process whereby sperm is placed into the vagina by means other than sexual intercourse

basal body temperature — the temperature of the body at rest (one hour)

Basic Infertile Pattern — several consecutive days where the infertile cervical mucus remains the same consistency (whether it be dry, flaky, sticky or thick).

BBT — Basal Body Temperature

BIP — Basic Infertile Pattern

Billings method — also known as the ovulation method, a means to determine ovulation by reading changes in cervical mucus

bladder — a membranous sac that holds urine until it is passed through the urethra out of the body

blastocyst — a ball of cells arranged in an inner and outer layer surrounding a fluid, resulting from cell division of a fertilized egg; a fertilized egg between the stages of a zygote and an embryo,

three to four days after fertilization and before
uterine implantation

breech birth — when a baby is delivered vaginally in any
position other than head first

carrier — a person who has a recessive gene for a genetic trait (often a disease) that does not manifest
itself physically

cervical crypts — chambers in the cervix that produce
different types of mucus

cervix — the lower portion of the uterus, which
is shaped like a neck

chromosome — a rod-shaped body inside a cell,
composed of hundreds of genes, which
contains instructions for producing a new
cell with the same characteristics as the
parent cell

clitoris — part of the external female genitalia, a sensitive
organ containing erectile tissue, located above
the urethra

CM — cervical mucus

corpus luteum — Latin for yellow body, the empty
ovarian follicle that turns yellow and secretes
estrogen and large amounts of progesterone for
12 to 16 days

Cowper's glands — small, pea-shaped glands that
secrete an alkaline fluid, located below the
prostate

dilation — the expanding of an opening; the first stage in
labor, in which the cervix widens, or opens, for
the fetus to pass through

DNA — deoxyribonucleic acid, a molecule that carries
the genetic material that determines the inherited
characterstics of an organism

dominant gene — one gene of a pair that whenever

present displays its characteristics

douche — a jet of water applied to the body internally, especially the vagina, for cleaning or medical purposes

ectopic pregnancy — the abnormal implantation of the embryo in one of the fallopian tubes instead of the uterus

ejaculation — the emission of semen during the male orgasm

embryo — a fertilized egg implanted in the uterus during the first three months of pregnancy

endometrium — the lining of the uterus

epididymis — a tightly coiled tube that stores sperm and secretes a small amount of seminal fluid; sperm pass through this tube

erection — the swelling and hardening of the penis as it is engorged with blood

estrogen — the female sex hormone produced by the ovaries

expulsion — the second stage in labor, in which the fetus is forcibly pushed out of the uterus

fallopian tubes — the ducts on either side of the uterus through which the egg is carried from the ovaries

false high rise — a rise in the BBT temperature above the coverline, followed by a drop below the coverline (instead of remaining higher several days); indicates ovulation may not have occurred

fertilization — the union of the male and female sex cells (sperm and egg) to produce a one-celled individual called a zygote

fetus — the eight to nine-week-old embryo after developing bone cells; the name of the developing child during approximately the last six months of a nine-month pregnancy

fimbriae — the finger-like projections at the end of the fallopian tubes that "catch" the released egg

follicle — the layers of cells enveloping the egg

fraternal twins — two eggs, fertilized by two sperm, that develop at the same time in the uterus

G-type mucus — an infertile, pasty, barrier mucus that is opaque and sticky or crumbly; forms an impenetrable barrier to sperm

gene — a segment of DNA that encodes specific traits; a piece of genetic information on a chromosome

gestation — the period during which the embryo/fetus develops in the uterus

gland — an organ in the body that secretes chemical compounds called hormones

heredity — the passing-on of genetic traits from parents to their offspring

hormone — a chemical compound released from specific glands to control particular body functions

implantation — the process by which the blastocyst attaches itself to the wall of the uterus

L-type mucus — infertile, beaded mucus, of a thick, lumpy texture; a sign of the start of fertility

labia — Latin for "large lips", the folds of skin enclosing the female external genitalia

labor — the process of birth resulting from the rhythmic and forceful contractions of the uterus: dilation, expulsion and the placental stage

luteinizing hormone — released from the pituitary gland, a chemical that promotes the production of egg cells by the ovaries and the development of the corpus luteum

menstruation — the periodic discharge of blood, mucus and tissue comprising the endometrium, or lining, of the uterus

mitosis — cell division resulting in two cells, each identical new cell containing identical genetic material as the parent cell

mittelschmerz — a German term for the abdominal pain that may occur in the middle of a menstrual cycle, signifying ovulation either has happened or is about to happen

monophasic cycle — a menstrual cycle in which ovulation does not occur (also called anovulatory)

mons pubis — skin and hair-covered padding of fat over a bone called the symphysis pubic

nucleus — the center of a cell where genetic information is stored; the head of a sperm that has penetrated the egg and dropped off its tail

os — Latin for "opening"

os diameter — the size of an opening

ovary — one of the two almond-shaped female sex glands located on either side of the uterus, containing a woman's eggs

ovulation — the release of the egg(s) from the ovary

ovum/ova — egg/eggs

oxytocin — a hormone that stimulates the uterus to contract and open the birth canal

Peak day — the last day the cervical mucus presents one or more fertile signs

penis — the male copulatory organ composed of spongy, erectile tissue, through which semen and urine travel

perineum — the skin-covered, muscular region between the external genitalia and the anus

placenta — an organ attached to the wall of the uterus that absorbs oxygen and nutrients from the mother's blood and removes waste products from the blood of the fetus

post-ovulatory phase — the phase in the menstrual cycle beginning after ovulation and continuing until the start of the next cycle (first day of menstruation, or bleeding)

pre-ovulatory phase — the phase in the menstrual cycle beginning the first day of the cycle (the first day of menstruation, or bleeding) and ending at the time of ovulation

pregnant — having an embryo or fetus developing inside the uterus

progesterone — secreted by the corpus luteum, a hormone that changes the nature of the fertile mucus and maintains the lining of the uterus

prostate gland — a gland in males that secretes the thin, alkaline substance that makes up the largest part of seminal fluid

recessive gene — a gene that exhibits its characteristics only when the dominant gene is not present

S-type mucus — fertile cervical mucus that is clear and stretchy, resembling raw egg white

scrotum — the sac of skin beneath the penis that holds the testes

semen — a mixture of seminal fluid and sperm stored in the seminal vesicles and ejaculated

seminiferous tubules — small tubes in the testes where sperm are produced

seminal vesicles — pouches which produce and release seminal fluid

seminal fluid — a thick milky liquid containing nutrients to support the sperm and enhance their motility

sexual intercourse — genital contact between individuals, especially the placing of a man's penis inside a woman's vagina

sperm — the male reproductive cell made up of a head, a midpiece and a tail

spermatogenesis — the production and maturation of sperm

sperm motility — a sperm's ability to move (at least 40

percent of a man's sperm should be active to
ensure fertility)

temperature shift (thermal shift) — a change in the basal
body temperature from a period of low
temperatures to a set of higher temperatures; can
indicate that ovulation has occurred

testes — two small male sexual glands that produce
sperm

testosterone — the primary male sex hormone, which
causes the male secondary sex characteristics

trimester — one of the three-month blocks of time in a
pregnancy

ultrasound — a diagnostic procedure whereby high
frequency sound waves, transmitted into the
body, bounce off tissues of different densities and
are recorded, creating an image on a computer
monitor

urethra — the tube that carries urine from the bladder to
the outside of the body

uterus — the female organ in which the embryo/fetus
develops; the womb

vagina — the expandable canal leading from the outside
of the female genitalia to the cervix of the uterus

vas deferens — ducts that transfer sperm from the testes
to the outside of the body

vulva — the outside parts of the female reproductive
organs

zygote — the new cell formed by the process of
fertilization

Appendix A
The Diet Theory

Because couples are looking for all the information they can find to make an educated choice, I decided to include the diet information in this book. The theory behind the diet is that a woman's consumption of certain foods and avoidance of others will cause a chemical change within her, resulting in conditions more favorable for conceiving a child of a particular sex. I am skeptical about using diet to preselect the sex of a baby. I believe that relying on the normal functioning of the female body is enough to increase one's chances. Using a diet method means following a rigorous schedule of dietary restrictions that I and many other medical professionals believe are not beneficial to a woman who is trying to conceive.

Hazel Chesterman-Phillips discusses her thoughts on the diet theory in her 1997 book, *Choose the Sex of Your Baby—The Natural Way*. Her feelings and mine seem to concur. In her book she relates how the diet works. A French gynecologist by the name of Dr. Papa determined how to conceive a boy or girl based on the four mineral salts found within the body. He surmised that to conceive a boy, there needs be an increase in sodium and potassium. These two alkalis attract the male sperm. To conceive a girl, calcium and magnesium are the salts required as they attract the female sperm. If the chemical composition of the egg were altered, it would attract the desired sperm.

What follows is a list of the foods recommended by the diet theory to help conceive a boy or a girl. Please do not start either of these diets without medical supervision. The high-salt "boy diet" would be dangerous for a woman with high blood pressure. Similarly, the high-calcium "girl" diet would be dangerous for a woman with a high calcium level or with kidney stones. I implore you to compare this diet with the Canada Food Guide or the Dietary Guidelines for Americans to see where the sex preselection diets are lacking valuable nutrients. The Canadian and U.S. guidelines can be found by searching the Health Canda Web site, *www.hc-sc.gc.ca*, and the United States Food and Drug Administration Web site, *www.fda.gov*, respectively. These two government guides are the only diets I recommend!

Trying for a Boy
The purpose is to increase the levels of sodium and potassium.

The foods permitted are

- Tea and coffee—rich in potassium
- Alcohol—wine is high in potassium, beer has sodium and potassium
- All meats, all fish (high in both) and two eggs per week
- All fresh or dried fruit, especially bananas, that are rich in potassium
- Most vegetables
- Soups, pickles, olives
- Pasta and rice

The foods contraindicated are

- Milk products—no milk, cheese, yogurt

- Shellfish, molluscs
- Salad vegetables—raw cauliflower, spinach, cabbage
- Mustard, nuts, cocoa, chocolate

Trying for a Girl

The foods permitted are

- Milk, milk, milk—as much as you can drink—750 milliliters/25 ounces per day but not more than 2 liters/roughly half a gallon per day
- Yogurt, unsalted butter, cheese
- Only fresh or frozen apples, pears, clementines, strawberries and raspberries, not more than 150 grams/roughly 5 ounces per day
- Eggs
- Unsalted or unleavened bread
- Rice and pasta
- Unsalted nuts
- Small amounts of potatoes, fresh or frozen carrots, peas, green beans, onions, leaks, turnips
- Canned pineapples, peaches and plums, not packed in syrup
- Only 125 grams/roughly 1 ounce of meat or fish per day

The foods contraindicated are

- Salt and all salted foods
- Coffee, tea, soda pop
- Wine, beer, cider, liquors
- Fruit loaves, buns
- Shellfish
- Chocolate and sweets

- All fresh fruit except those listed as permitted—no dried fruit
- Parsley, spinach, mushrooms, fennel, avocados, tomatoes, cauliflower, cabbage, dried peas, beans
- All premade meals and sauces

Appendix B
Answers to Practice Chart

1. Determine the length of the cycle: 29 days.

2. Temperature Chart
a) Determine the day of the shift. Count the first six low temperatures and draw a coverline above the highest dot. Count three high temperatures. Draw a vertical line between the last low temperature and the first high temperature and extend the line straight up past the top line, "Day of Month": the coverline is drawn between 36.8 °C and 36.9 °C; the vertical line is drawn down between day 16 and day 17 (May 21 and 22); the shift in temperature occurs on day 22 (May 17).

b) Check for factors (stress, illness, medications, sleep problems) that may influence the temperature: she was up at 5:00 a.m. on day 6 (May 11).

c) Identify the first day of the post-ovulatory infertile phase: day 22 (May 17).

3. Mucus Pattern
a) Determine the length of her period: five days.

b) Identify the first appearance of mucus: day 13 (May 8).

c) Identify the pre-ovulatory infertile phase. Look for the Basic Infertile Pattern (BIP) of non-changing mucus, or dry, flaky mucus and/or dry vaginal sensations: The pre-ovulatory phase is from day 1 to day 8

(May 6 to May 13). [*Note: the menstrual days are included in the infertile phase because they were followed by dry days. If you are trying to prevent a pregnancy, either refrain from intercourse or use a non-lubricated condom, until you are certain you are in the BIP. Remember, the early infertile days are those before any mucus change occurs. The days may be dry or they may have a non-changing mucus pattern, e.g., flaky or sticky mucus and the sticky vaginal sensation. If the woman had experienced flaky mucus day after day, it would have been included in the infertile phase which would have been longer.*]

d) Identify the fertile phase, days of wet mucus, especially stretchy mucus. Mark the Peak day with an X. Number 1,2,3,4 on the four days after the Peak day: the fertile phase is from day 9 to day 19 (May 14 to May 24) inclusive; the Peak day is on day 15 (May 20); the numbers 1,2,3,4 would be on days 16, 17, 18, 19, respectively.

e) Identify the post-ovulatory infertile phase: day 20 (May 25).

f) Correspond the temperature chart with the mucus chart to identify the probable day of ovulation: day 21 (May 16).

4. Changes in Cervix
a) Identify the infertile phase (low, firm, closed, tilted): the infertile phase is from day 6 to day 8 (May 11 to 13); her cervix seemed higher on May 14, which shows the shift to more fertile days.

b) Identify the fertile phase (high, soft, open, straight): The fertile phase is from day 8 to day 19 (May 14 to May 24). [*Note: not all signs of fertility may be present at one time.*

Having all signs present assures *fertility, but one or more signs* warns *that you may be fertile.*]

5. Other Indicators—identify other signs such as abdominal pain, et cetera, to determine ovulation: her breasts were sore on day 14 and day 15 (May 19 and 20); she experienced abdominal pain on day 21 (May 16).

Appendix C Fertility Chart

Please note: for Fahrenheit, your chart should begin with 96.9°F and end with 99.1°F, increasing in increments of a tenth of a degree.

Months _____

Day of Month																														1
Day of Cycle																														2
C M **Appearance**																														3
Sensation																														4
C e r v i x **Open/closed**																														5
Firm/soft																														6
Tilt																														7
Temperature °C																														8
37.3																														
37.2																														
37.1																														
37.0																														
36.9																														
B B T 36.8																														
36.7																														
36.6																														9
36.5																														
36.4																														
36.3																														
36.2																														
36.1																														
Intercourse																														10
Disturbances																														11
Other signs																														12

Mucus: Appearance — Period = **P** Flakey = **F** Sticky = **S** Dry = D L-type mucus = M Stretchy, Slippery = Ⓜ Peak = **X**
Sensation — Dry = **D** Sticky = **S** Wet = **W**
Cervix: Open = ○ Closed = ● Firm = **F** Soft = **S** Straight = I Titled = / High, medium, low = ● ˙ ● ˙ ○ ●
Other signs: Abdominal pain = **AP**